Intestinal Ills

by Alcinous Burton Jamison

TO THE UNFORTUNATE SUFFERER FROM ILLS DESCRIBED IN THIS VOLUME AND TO THOSE WHOM I HAVE HAD THE PLEASURE OF CURING THIS BOOK IS RESPECTFULLY DEDICATED

BEAUTY'S FALL.

It was an image good to see, With spirits high and full of glee, And robust health endowed; Its face was loveliness untold, Its lines were cast in beauty's mold; At its own shrine it bowed.

With perfect form in each respect, It proudly stood with head erect And skin surpassing fair; Surveyed itself from foot to head, And then complacently it said: "Naught can with me compare."

When lo the face began to pale, The body looked too thin and frail, The cheek had lost its glow; The tongue a tale of woe did tell, With nerves impaired its spirits fell; The fire of life burned low.

In the intestinal canal Waste matter lay, and sad to tell, Was left from day to day; And while it was neglected there It undermined that structure fair, And caused it to decay.

The doctor's words I would recall Who said: "Neglect precedes a fall," And verily 'tis true; For ye who disregard your health, And value not that precious wealth, Will surely live to rue.

PREFACE.

The following chapters were contributions to Health--a monthly magazine published in New York City. Certain peculiarities of form and considerable repetition of statement--both of which the reader cannot fail to notice--are owing to the fact that about two-thirds of the chapters were written under the caption "Auto-genetic Poisons in the Intestinal Canal and their Auto-infection." In revising these contributions for book form I have given to each chapter a caption of its leading thought; but I am convinced that repetition of some of the matters treated, especially if the repetition be in a somewhat different connection, is not such a very bad thing. I have used my blue pencil sparingly, and as a consequence the consecutive reader will find that constipation, diarrhea, biliousness, indigestion, auto-infection and proctitis are treated in nearly all the chapters--but with varying applications. Therefore anyone suffering from one of these complaints would better read the whole book instead of only the chapter with the corresponding title.

These pages were written for intelligent laymen by a specialist, during a busy, assiduous practice. I take such radical ground, however, going to the very root of the matter, that the general practitioner will do well to give my thesis his careful consideration; he should at least glance at the following Introduction for the gist of my claim.

CONTENTS.

* CHAPTER I.

MAN, COMPOSED ALMOST WHOLLY OF WATER, IS CONSTIPATED. WHY?

* CHAPTER II.

THE PHYSICS OF DIGESTION AND EGESTION

* CHAPTER III.

THE INTERDEPENDENCE OF ANUS, RECTUM, SIGMOID FLEXURE AND COLON

* CHAPTER IV.

INDIGESTION, INTESTINAL GAS AND OTHER MATTERS

* CHAPTER V.

KEY TO AUTO-INFECTION

* CHAPTER VI.

HOW AUTO-INFECTION AFFECTS THE GASTRIC DIGESTION, AND VICE VERSA

* CHAPTER VII.

HOW AUTO-INFECTION AFFECTS INTESTINAL DIGESTION, AND VICE VERSA

* CHAPTER VIII.

THE CAUSE OF CONSTIPATION AND HOW WE IGNORANTLY TREAT IT

* CHAPTER IX.

CURES FOR CONSTIPATION: "FEARFULLY AND WONDERFULLY MADE"

* CHAPTER X.

BILIOUSNESS AND BILIOUS ATTACKS

* CHAPTER XI.

KING LIVER AND BILE-BOUNCERS

* CHAPTER XII.

SEMI-CONSTIPATION AND ITS DANGERS

* CHAPTER XIII.

THE ETIOLOGY OF THE MOST COMMON FORM OF DIARRHEA, i.e., EXCESSIVE INTESTINAL PERISTALSIS

* CHAPTER XIV.

BALLOONING OF THE RECTUM

* CHAPTER XV.

BALLOONING OF THE RECTUM--continued

* CHAPTER XVI.

THE USUAL DIAGNOSIS AND TREATMENT OF BOWEL TROUBLES WRONG

* CHAPTER XVII.

COSTIVENESS

* CHAPTER XVIII.

INFLAMMATION

* CHAPTER XIX.

PROCTITIS AND PILES

* CHAPTER XX.

PRURITUS OR ITCHING OF THE ANUS

* CHAPTER XXI.

ABSCESS AND FISTULA

* CHAPTER XXII.

THE ORIGIN AND USE OF THE ENEMA

* CHAPTER XXIII.

HOW OFTEN SHOULD AN ENEMA BE TAKEN?

* CHAPTER XXIV.

MAN'S BEST FRIEND

* CHAPTER XXV.

PHYSIOLOGICAL IRRIGATION

* CHAPTER XXVI.

PROPER TREATMENT FOR DISEASES OF ANUS AND RECTUM ESSENTIAL

* CHAPTER XXVII.

THE BODY'S BOOK-KEEPING

* CHAPTER XXVIII.

SELECTION AND PREPARATION OF FOOD

* CHAPTER XXIX.

DIET FOR INDIGESTION

* CHAPTER XXX.

DIET FOR CONSTIPATION AND OBSTIPATION

* CHAPTER XXXI.

COSTIVENESS, DIET, ETC.

* CHAPTER XXXII.

DIET FOR DIARRHEA

A FINAL WORD

NO. 1.

CHRONIC CONSTIPATION AND THE USE OF THE ENEMA

NO. 2.

OBJECTIONS TO THE USE OF ENEMA ANSWERED

INTRODUCTION.

The keynote of this book is Proctitis, inflammation of the anal and rectal canals. Hardly a civilized man escapes proctitis from the day of the diaper to that of death. The diaper is in truth chiefly responsible for proctitis, and proctitis is in turn chiefly responsible for chronic constipation, chronic diarrhea, auto-infection; and hence for mal-assimilation, mal-nutrition, anemia; and for a thousand and one reflex functional derangements of the system as well. The inflamed surface of the intestinal canal (proctitis) inhibits the passage of feces. Absorbent glands begin to act on the retained sewage, and the whole system becomes more or less infected with poisonous bacteria. Various organs (especially the feeblest) endeavor to perform vicarious defecation, and the patient, the friends, and even the physician are deceived by such vicarious performance into thinking and treating it as a local ailment. I cannot, accordingly, insist too emphatically that proctitis, the exciting cause, must be treated primarily if we would cure chronic constipation. Millions of human beings are sent to untimely graves by these ailments. Indeed, the body of nearly every human being is a pest-house of absorbed poison instead of being the worthy temple of a wondrous soul. All due to Proctitis!

INTESTINAL ILLS

CHAPTER I.

MAN, COMPOSED ALMOST WHOLLY OF WATER, IS CONSTIPATED. WHY?

Naturally the mind of man was first educated to observe external objects and forces in their effects upon himself, and the external still continues to engross his attention as if he were a child in a kindergarten. Fascinated by the

Without, he ignores the Within. But, marvel of marvels, Disease (which when looked at with discerning eyes is seen to be an angel in disguise) comes to enlighten him concerning the world within. Disease gradually acquaints him with the fact that there are within him organs and functions corresponding to the objects and forces in the world without,--servitors in fact which must not be ignored under penalty of transforming them into foes to his well-being. Disease makes him aware that by ignoring the claims of his inner relations he has been converting his very food, juices and gases into insidious and formidable poisons, which perforce he absorbs into his blood and tissues and circulates throughout his entire system. Thus does the disguised angel admonish the ignorant that the rights of the inner world must not be ignored--that one's duties thereto cannot be neglected without disastrous consequences.

Thus does Pathology, which is really Physiology reversed, become the self-revealer par excellence. Through digestion and assimilation the physiological process takes up the food, juices and gases, to support and augment the life of man. The pathological process, on the contrary, because the conditions for nutrition are ignored, reverses the upbuilding processes; and the organs of life wither, waste and weaken, until life goes out like fire unfed.

Man has been slowly learning to take sanitary measures in reference to everything that contributes to comfort in his surroundings, and hygienic measures in reference to everything conducive to stability in his health.

Through ages he has learned, by experience and experiment, of the changes that inevitably occur in such perishable nutritive substances as water, milk, meats, vegetables, fruits, etc., if they be left uncared for; and he has been led thus to the inference of the law of decomposition--or putrefactive and fermentative changes. Idle substances, like idle minds, have decomposition and the devil for companions. Substances confined in containers open to the air--ponds, cesspools, etc.--are every-day object lessons to man of the fact that the chemical changes they undergo furnish the conditions for breeding bacterial poisons, and that these poisons are a dread menace to animal life.

If the reader will observe the analogy between the decomposition of substances in vessels or pools, and the decomposition of food in the reservoir called the stomach; and its further decomposition in a long canal (the small intestine), connecting the stomach with other receptacles called the colon and sigmoid flexure; and then the decomposition of their contents; he will readily comprehend the chemical putrefactive or fermentative changes or bacterial action that take place in the organism, if for any reason the contents be confined.

Of the four chief elements that enter into the composition of living bodies three are gaseous, or convertible into gas. In the physical man water constitutes three-fourths of the weight of the body. This being so we realize why, notwithstanding our sense of solidity and weight, chemical changes occur quite as readily in our organism as in the substances we see about us. There are no waterproof walls in the body of man to impede the percolation of liquids freighted with promiscuous Passengers from the alimentary canal; Passengers designed to nourish the organs for which they have an affinity. But there are those that have no organic affinity, and these are tramps, vagabonds, and even murderers, disturbing and destroying the normal functions of the system. Through extravasation, that is, through fluid infiltration of tissues, these Passengers come to be one with us, and we make them part of our tissue; but some of the Passengers are the demolishers of the living temple.

Water is universally present in all the tissues of the body, and it is indispensable for introducing new substances into the system and for eliminating the worn-out tissues and foreign substances. It is indeed important to emphasize the fact that properly to eliminate the foreign and waste products from the system requires, in a healthy person, at least five pints of water during twenty-four hours.

The amount of gastric juice secreted in twenty-four hours is from six to fourteen pints; of pancreatic juice, one pint; of bile there are two to three pints, and of saliva one to three pints. It is estimated that the juices secreted during digestion in a man weighing 140 pounds amount to twenty-three pounds in twenty-four hours. These fluids are poured back and forth in the process of transforming food into flesh and eliminating waste material.

In the alimentary canal there are vessels for holding fluid, semi-fluid and moist masses of substance, in all of which decomposition occurs if the substances be retained beyond the normal length of time. These vessels or reservoirs are the stomach, duodenum, small intestines, colon, sigmoid flexure, and too often the rectum. Through the harmonious action of this intestinal retinue of servitors man is well equipped and qualified for health, and he in whom this harmonious subservience prevails is among the blessed and elect of mankind. But alas! the great majority of human beings are sufferers from the inharmonious and insubordinate action of these servitors. How many a human being suffers from chronic constipation and indigestion, the exciting causes of which are insidious, and the consequences a protean enemy to his happiness! Medical writers on the subject of chronic constipation have assigned numerous causes, and likewise prescribed multitudinous remedies to the patient; but as a general rule this patient, after suffering various woes, if still surviving the many years of medication, rebels against taking further remedies and resigns himself to the chronic enemy on the best terms he can make with diet.

For this large class of chronic sufferers we have good news; and for the class that have suffered five or ten years we have better news; and for the class of infants and children that have started on the road of ill-health we have real glad tidings. To know that there is only one chief cause for chronic constipation and its train of disorders, and that that cause overshadows all other causes combined, and is easily diagnosed and treated, is news long hoped and prayed for by a multitude of sufferers the world over.

Twenty years as a specialist in diseases of the lower bowels have demonstrated to the writer that chronic inflammation, and often ulceration, of the rectum and sigmoid flexure, in ninety-nine cases out of a hundred, is the cause of chronic constipation and the long army of ills resulting from it. And yet, as the reader is well aware, constipation has had many "causes," since the days of Hippocrates, especially the abnormal condition of the liver.

The etiology, that is, the exciting cause, of the inflammation of the anus, rectum, colon, etc., may date from the time a diaper was placed on the new-born infant. Excoriations of the integument about the anus by the excretions of bowels and bladder indicate that the mucous membrane of anus and rectum demands local remedies, as well as the integument of the buttocks, and that it is not the liver which is at fault. The many applications of the diaper during the period of its use, and the frequently delayed removal at night or during long rides in baby wagons, railway trains or carriages, and during long social visits of the nurse; constipating foods, lack of drinking water, constipating medicines, followed by all sorts of purgatives, etc., are among a few of the direct causes of diseases of the rectum. A child at the age of eighteen months with a healthy rectum is most rare.

The ten thousand and one chances for contracting disease of the anus and rectum do not cease with the period of infancy. The child is left pretty much to shift for itself as to regularity of eating and the evacuation of the contents of its bowels, wherein disease has already obtained a foothold. All kinds of foodstuffs, at all hours, with seeds, stones, etc., are poked into its stomach, followed by constipating remedies to quiet inevitable troubles, or brisk purgatives given with the hope of expelling the arrested contents of the bowels. Is it any wonder that ninety-eight persons of adult age out of every hundred suffer more or less from chronic inflammation and ulceration of anus, rectum, sigmoid flexure, colon, or appendix?

Traumatic (externally produced) injuries to the mucous membrane of the rectum frequently cause inflammation, and hard pieces of bone, wood, seeds, imbedded in the feces, scratch, cut and bruise the tissues before and during the act of defecation. Cold boards, stones, earth and other substances used as seats may produce inflammation of the rectum. There are many and various causes which may be the means of exciting inflammation of the anus and rectum later in life; but it is the writer's opinion that the cause can be traced back to infancy or early childhood, and that accidents or imprudence in after years merely excite an already-existing chronic inflammation. Piles, fissure, itching pockets, tabs, prolapse, abscesses, fistul? etc., are only the outcome and symptoms of a chronic disease which has incubated for fifteen, twenty or more years. None of this list of troubles produces constipation. It is the inflammation located at the middle portion of the rectum and extending into the sigmoid flexure that causes constipation; that protean monster which deranges more lives with nervousness than any other pathological condition to which the flesh of man is heir!

CHAPTER II.

THE PHYSICS OF DIGESTION AND EGESTION.

A tree is simply an extension from its roots; and, in an analogous manner, man's body may be said to be an extension from the alimentary canal. Does it not follow, consequently, that the digestive apparatus, from a physiological point of view, is the most important organ of the human body? It must be prime and paramount because all other organs depend upon it: it provides them with nourishment for preservation and improvement, and it punishes them--if they do not mind the laws of normality--by withholding its gifts, or by presenting these gifts in the form of poisons that impoverish, hinder and degenerate the system of organs. Uncleanliness is surely one of the chief ways in which physiological thoughtlessness is exhibited, and due punishment will inevitably follow disobedience.

Foodstuffs are prepared for assimilation in the alimentary laboratory through the process of normal fermentation. Is it not essential, therefore, that the connecting canals and receptacles be cleansed of the fermented debris that may remain unused and unexpelled, before more food be taken by the digestive apparatus? The all-important question is:--How soon and how well have the residuary part of the food (for some part will always be undigested or unassimilated), and the waste resulting from worn-out tissues of the various organs, been eliminated from the system? Wisdom declares that it is not so much what we eat, but what and how well we eliminate, that decides the issues of health and disease. Do the egesta pass out in the form of normal feces? Three times in twenty-four hours foodstuffs are taken, and as many times the bowels should be freed of accumulated excrement and gases. Does Nature have her way, or do neglect and bad habits rule the assimilative and eliminative functions of the bowels?

The habit of storing feces for twenty-four hours ought to concur and keep pace with a habit of eating one meal in the same period. Household and laboratory receptacles in which fermentation has occurred are emptied and cleaned before fresh material is put into them. Is not the same precaution more essential with the receptacles for digestion and egestion? They constitute our chief physiological economy; they are precious household and laboratory utensils; exceedingly precious, as we can purchase no other set when these are worn and wasted beyond repair. What marvelous possessions, and how reckless most of us are with them! Neither love nor money will bring another "body"-house to us when this decays; when poisons or parasites infest it as the result of a pernicious diathesis, of debasing, destructive tendencies; in short, of unmindfulness!

Too often criminal negligence or the lack of proper convenience has brought on the habit of using the intestinal canal as a storehouse for dried feces, and the glands and blood-vessels as reservoirs for the absorbed fluid poisons from the feces that have been stored and thus dried. This baneful habit is general throughout civilized communities. It is this habit that has made the words "constipation," "indigestion," "diarrhea," etc., familiar and household subjects of complaint. Medical writers agree that "constipation" is the most common malady that afflicts mankind; but they are also unanimous in preposterously attributing the cause to the abnormal action of the liver and the secondary symptoms of constipation.

Chronic constipation is the result of proctitis and colitis. Proctitis, the inflammation of the rectal and anal canals, is the most common disease that afflicts the human creature from infancy to old age; and colitis is only the extension of proctitis to the colon.

The scientific diagnosis of constipation predicates proctitis and sometimes colitis. It is declared that constipation is its primary symptom; and that diarrhea is one of its secondary symptoms, resulting from constipation. There is a legion of secondary symptoms of proctitis, all of which medical empiricism considers and denominates causes. As constipation is such an every-day complaint of almost everybody one meets, it will not tax our imagination unduly to conceive how it may be a frequent cause of diarrhea, which is only Nature's effort to get rid of its useless and excessive burden of retained feces and gases. Constipation, semi-constipation, and irregular action of the bowels, excessive fermentation, putrefaction, self-generated or auto-infection, are the factors to be considered. It is to be noted that in many cases diarrhea is simply an increased peristalsis of the bowels, often due to local and diffused irritation and often to inflammation of the mucous membrane (not infrequently with ulceration); all of these may be the outcome of fecal impaction.

To make intelligible the physics of the digestive and egestive processes, we must understand the apparatus. One would naturally think that were the bends or curves of the large intestine undone, it would be found to be a long, straight, smooth canal or bore like a rubber tube. But such is not the case. The outer muscular longitudinal bands are much shorter than the musculo-areolo-mucous tube, an arrangement which brings about a transverse puckering of the gut and mucous membrane, thus forming valves, folds, sacs or pouches at short intervals along the canal. These transverse folds or valves inhibit the too hasty passage of the feces along the bowels by checking and retaining the egested product in the large recesses or pools between the folds; they thus serve as so many dams in the passage of feces toward elimination. This wise provision of Nature to moderate the steady motion of the feces as they proceed toward the sigmoid flexure or receptacle, to wait there till there is a proper stimulus for expulsion, is wofully abused by man. He is quite willing to take foodstuffs three or four times a day, to fill the long row of intestinal pools between the dams with feces and gases in all stages of decomposition, not dreaming of the danger from developing bacteria and their absorption into the system.

Really he is inclined to eat at all times, yet begrudges a few minutes spent in a hurried effort to perform the act of defecation once in twenty-four hours. Some of us even have our minds absorbed in reading while awaiting an "automatic action" of the bowels. What a contrast between the gusto and time spent in taking foodstuffs and the indifference and indolence regarding the action of the bowels, unless indeed severe biliousness or diarrhea reminds us strongly of our sewer of waste products.

An attack of acute or chronic diarrhea is the penalty some pay for long inattention to the demands nature makes for intestinal cleanliness three times in twenty-four hours. Constipated people, semi-constipated people, irregular people and twenty-four-hour people, are not healthy. They are constantly being poisoned by the abnormal products of indigestion and putrefaction resulting from fecal stagnation, which products enter the blood and circulate through every tissue of the body.

All cases of proctitis are more or less accompanied by constipation and diarrhea. In all cases of chronic constipation I have found proctitis, and often colitis, and am forced to believe it is the most common and proximate cause of chronic constipation of the bowels. Constipation being a primary symptom, there must of necessity follow numerous secondary symptoms, of which diarrhea well marks the progress of septic infection. Some of the symptoms of infection are headache, megrim, vertigo, dyspepsia, foul tongue and mouth, back-aches, stiff neck, gnawing pain or numb feeling at the lower end of the spine, biliousness, bad odor from breath and skin, muddy complexion, cold hands and feet, jaundice, neurasthenia, loss of memory, drowsy feeling, pernicious anemia, emaciation, flabby obesity with pallor, capricious appetite, fits of great mental depression, palpitation of the heart, bloating of the stomach and bowels, disturbance of the kidneys, liver, lungs and mucous membrane in general, and especially chronic rhinitis and pharyngitis, which latter are among the first symptoms of imperfect alimentary excretion.

As auto-intoxication (that condition of the system when it is continually poisoned, usually by one's own excretions) gains the mastery of the vital forces at any period of life, the mucous membranes are likely to be first affected by inflammation of catarrhal character; then the serous membranes of the body. Mal-assimilation, mal-nutrition, cell-atrophy, are symptoms of the giving way of the vital energies to the invasion of the filth and bacterial poisons absorbed from the intestinal canal.

On the inner surface of the alimentary canal, from the stomach to the colon, there are, it is estimated, over 20,000,000 rootlets (called glands, lacteals, follicles, villi), which take up intestinal juices as roots of a plant take sap from the soil. These millions of rootlets give a velvety appearance to the alimentary canal, like a nap or downy surface. Intestinal rootlets of the small intestines, like vegetal rootlets, demand a certain amount of normal fluid and solid substance, free from noxious gas. It is the down or nap of fabrics, and not their body, that shows damage first. So it is with the frail structure of vegetal and animal life if not properly supplied with nourishment from day to day. There is probably in the vegetal bodies a continuous circulation of sap corresponding to the digestive circulating fluids of the alimentary canal. This circulation from the alimentary canal to the blood-vessels, and from the blood-vessels to the alimentary canal, involves a wonderful mechanism, facilitating the flow of several gallons daily from each to the other during the process of metamorphosis of food into flesh. You can thus see how inevitable it is that the functions of these millions of secreting and excreting rootlets will be disturbed by the clogging of the system with filth and bacterial poisons as a consequence of chronic constipation, biliousness and general foulness of the alimentary canal. Through such disturbance nutrition is diminished, cell-atrophy progresses, and emaciation becomes more marked. The progressive destruction of these rootlets, involving the pathological change indicated, will be manifest in one of its results, either costiveness or diarrhea.

Often the power of properly digesting and absorbing the foodstuffs is so greatly diminished that the alimentary canal is about as useless as a soft rubber tube. Millions on millions of these glands, lacteals and follicles in the stomach and small intestines, are destroyed like the rootlets of a plant or tree in unwholesome soil. The active circulation of the digestive fluids ceases, and the sufferer is said to be costive or to have chronic diarrhea. Both symptoms are the outgrowth of many years of intestinal foulness, and indicate the degree and character of intestinal irritability and semi-starvation of the body, as a consequence of either the absorption of poisons or the excessive elimination of the vital substance of the body through diarrhea.

CHAPTER III.

THE INTER-DEPENDENCE OF ANUS, RECTUM, SIGMOID FLEXURE, AND COLON.

Physiologically, or in a normal state, the rectum is not a receptacle for liquids and feces but a conduit during the act of defecation. Should, therefore, the feces have passed into the rectum and the desire to stool be not responded to--though the desire continue urgent--the feces will be returned to the sigmoid cavity by physiological action. When, however, the functions of the anus and rectum are disturbed by chronic inflammation, etc., the lower portion of the rectum becomes a more or less roomy pouch, a receptacle for feces and liquids; and instead of being physiologically empty it becomes pathologically distended, the result of spasmodic action or of more or less permanent stricture of the sphincter ani. See illustration in my book entitled How to Become Strong (page 14).

The putrid fecal mass of solid and liquid contents accumulated in the artificial reservoir at the end of the intestinal sewer, is one of the most common and serious pathogenic (disease-producing) and pyogenic (pus-producing) sources, which, by auto-infection, afflict man from infancy to old age. Here--in the dilated and obstructed sewer--the ptomain and leucomain class of poisons, and many of the poisonous germs, led by the king of morbid disturbers, the bacillus coli communis, find another and last chance to be taken up by the absorbing cells of the mucous membrane and returned to the blood; with which they are carried to all parts of the body, clogging the glands, choking up the pores and obstructing the circulation, thereby causing congestion and inflammation of the various organs. The action of cathartics, laxatives, etc., fills the ano-rectal cavity with a watery solution of foul substances; this solution is readily absorbed into the circulation, aggravating the auto-intoxication (the established self-poisoned condition) already existing. Danger does not end with the absorption of bacterial poisons, as we have to reckon with the deleterious effects of the various intestinal gases, resulting, with rapid augmentation of volume, from the putrefactive changes in the imprisoned feculent matter.

A sphincter ani permanently constricted or irritable owing to disease results in an abnormal receptacle just above the anal orifice (as shown in the illustration referred to); and a constricted and irritable rectum results in the impaction and dilatation of the sigmoid cavity, which is normally a receptacle, closed at its lower end by circular fibres separating it (the cavity) from the rectum and performing the function of a sphincter muscle. The rectal muscular fibres perform the office of a sphincter for the sigmoid cavity. The pathological changes that result in rectal impaction of feces usually extend to the sigmoid cavity. This cavity is 17-1/2 inches in length, shaped in a double curve like an italic S. Civilized man should consider the disturbance to the functional action of body and brain, and the danger to health and longevity involved in the storage of effete and fetid matter. The disturbance and danger are enhanced when the tissues of the sigmoid flexure and the rectum are invaded by inflammation. A healthy action of the sigmoid receptacle depends on the rectum (a conduit six to eight inches in length); and as it is the universal verdict that disease of the rectum is one of the most common maladies that afflict the human race, it must inevitably follow that the feces will be abnormally stored in the sigmoid cavity, occasioning thereby habitual constipation which in turn brings on a host of functional disturbances throughout the system.

The colon is a receptacle and a conduit some three feet in length (see ib. p.

13) and its action depends upon the ability of the sigmoid flexure to perform its function as a final normal receptacle; and this in turn upon the rectum, which depends on the sphincter ani. The colon does not appear to possess any digestive powers, though it is capable of absorbing substances. Its function is not only to receive and forward the trifling residue of food which escapes digestion and absorption, but chiefly to excrete, through its own minute glands, the waste of the system coming from the blood.

The excretion from these glands of the colon into the colon, plus the effete portion of the food received by the colon from the small intestine, approximate in weight from four to six ounces in an adult person in twenty-four hours; and of this amount passed 75 per cent is water; so that were the excreta dried the solid matter thus evacuated would not be found to weigh more than one ounce, or one and a half ounces.

CHAPTER IV.

INDIGESTION, INTESTINAL GAS, AND OTHER MATTERS.

We noted the fact that the "digestive secretions" in a man weighing 140 pounds amount to twenty-three pounds in twenty-four hours; now add to these the food and liquids taken in that period, and you will form some estimate of the work done in the human chemical laboratory in its normal and abnormal states.

We noted further that substances confined too long in receptacles decompose and generate pathogenic poisons, that is, poisons productive of disease; and that the intestinal reservoirs are no exception to this law of putrefactive changes. How could we avoid drawing the inference, therefore, that disease-breeding germs, (generated in the organism and hence called "autogenetic"), and their auto-infection, i.e., absorption by the system, are an inevitable consequence of the undue retention and fermentation of the contents of these reservoirs: a consequence, in other words, of that intestinal uncleanliness commonly called biliousness, constipation, indigestion.

By far the most common and immediate source of autogenetic (self-produced) poisons and their auto-infection, is some degree of chronic constipation and the deadening, smothering effects of constipation on digestion; an effect analogous to what takes place when we allow waste material or ashes to bank up against a fire, shutting off its draft. Does the fire then continue to digest the coal? Clog up the receptacle for ashes and the coal grows cold. Dam up the colon or sigmoid and digestion is disturbed, diminished and debased, as evidenced by the local and general discomfort, and later by the train of inevitable disorders.

Indigestion is a household word. It has the widest range of all the diseases, because it forms a part of almost every other; and some diseases, such as chronic catarrh and pulmonary consumption, are in many cases produced by indigestion; which in turn had its source in chronic constipation caused by injury or inflammation of the lower bowel, as explained in our first chapter.

Diminished nutrition, impoverished blood, and loss of weight of from ten to twenty-five pounds, are the signs that indicate the coming disaster to the sufferer from auto-intoxication: the thoroughly poisoned state of the system resulting from auto-infection.

Vessels used by the dairyman and by those who furnish us with food products and liquids are kept scrupulously clean. Why? Because it is a question of loss of trade--of money. Should these vessels be used when foul from fermentation or putrefaction of their contents, Wealth would flee from the coffers of our purveyors, and the Boards of Health would, or rather should, take a hand in the matter. And these same purveyors, by the way, why do they care more for Wealth than for Health, their own and ours? But why are we all of us so neglectful of Inner cleanliness and so careful of Outer? The receptacles of the inner man reek with augean filth, and we cleanse them not. The immortal fountains of Health and Happiness are dammed, blasted and degraded by just this neglect of our imperative duty; the duty of furnishing full opportunity for the functions of replenishment and life, by keeping the sewer passages clear.

Are a sour stomach and foul intestinal canal fit receptacles for food and liquids? When our receptacles are in this condition, why do we add more material for the generation of poisons of the ptomain and leucomain classes, and morbid gaseous elements? It has been demonstrated that during fermentation an apple will evolve a volume of gas six hundred times its own size. What folly then to add to the fermenting mass! Food taken under such conditions will produce results not hard to imagine.

The gases that are commonly found in the stomach and small intestines are carbonic acid, nitrogen, oxygen and hydrogen; while, besides all these, sulphureted and carbureted hydrogen are found in the large intestine, causing in a normal state the necessary and useful distention of the alimentary canal. The writer has long regarded the abnormal production of gaseous substances in the intestinal canal from putrefactive changes as of itself not only a grave menace to health, but as a condition productive of morbific results of which we have still much to learn. The more or less constant and excessive distention of the whole or even of a part of the intestinal canal by gases is a serious condition, affecting as it does the various organs of the body, not only through the absorption of these gases into the general circulation but also through the reflex nervous reaction of these organs. It is astonishing what amount of mechanical force is exerted by the gases in the intestinal canal. They distend not only the muscular walls of the intestines and stomach but the strong abdominal walls as well, until the clothing worn has to be loosened for ease and comfort. This more or less extreme mechanical pressure may account for many cases of hernia, prolapse of the uterus, dislocation of various organs, disturbance of the circulation of the blood, and interference with the function of the nervous system, as indicated by its many protests in the way of aches and pains. Naval-constructor Hobson has lately demonstrated the dynamic power of gas confined in bags or receptacles in raising battleships; and it still remains for some physiologist or pathologist to demonstrate the morbid dynamic results of gases confined in the alimentary apparatus. The deleterious effect of the abnormal quantity of gases on all the organs of the body is imperfectly understood at present, but will be better apprehended when we are able to study more minutely the pathogenic poisons of the human system. It is known, however, that a stream of carbonic acid gas, or even of hydrogen, will paralyze a muscle against which it is directed.

CHAPTER V.

KEY TO AUTO-INFECTION.

In a previous chapter we stated that the average quantity of fecal discharge daily, by an adult, is from four to six ounces, and that of this weight 75 per cent is water. We referred of course to the daily passage from the bowels alone, not including that from the bladder.

Our studies have thus furnished us with the key wherewith to unlock the secret chambers of auto-infection. What is that key? It is the discovery that the system may possibly absorb as high as three-fourths of this feculent substance in the colon; that this absorption is made possible by an obstructed or sluggish intestinal canal where disease germs are propagated and lodged; that these germs, along with a certain amount of excrement, invade the tissues by absorption; and that we thus have the system constantly saturated with poisonous germs and filth, re-excreted, re-absorbed and re-secreted--no one knows how many times--by the various organs of the body.

That the importance of intestinal cleanliness may be better appreciated, I will quote from the following authors on the subjects of excretion, absorption and circulation of the intestinal fluids.

Dr. Murchison states that:

"From what is now known of the diffusibility of fluids through animal membranes, it is impossible to conceive bile long in contact with the lining membrane of the gall-bladder, bile-ducts, and intestine, without a portion of it (including the dissolved pigment) passing into the blood. A circulation is constantly taking place between the fluid contents of the bowel and the blood, the existence of which, till within the last few years, was quite unknown, and which even now is too little heeded. It is now known, says Dr. Parker, that in varying degrees there is a constant transit of fluid from the blood into the alimentary canal, and as rapid absorption. The amount thus poured out and absorbed in twenty-four hours is almost incredible, and of itself constitutes a secondary or intermediate circulation never dreamt of by Harvey. The amount of gastric juice alone passing into the stomach in a day, and then re-absorbed, amounted in the case lately examined by Grunewald to nearly 23 imperial pints. If we put it at 12 pints we shall certainly be within the mark. The pancreas, according to Krer, furnishes 12-1/2 pints in twenty-four hours, while the salivary glands pour out at least 3 pints in the same time. The amount of the bile is probably over 2 pints. The amount given out by the intestinal mucous membrane cannot be guessed at, but must be enormous. Altogether the amount of fluid effused into the alimentary canal in twenty-four hours amounts to much more than the whole amount of blood in the body (which is 18 pounds in a man weighing 143 pounds); in other words, every portion of the blood may, and possibly does, pass several times into the alimentary canal in twenty-four hours. The effect of this continual out-pouring is supposed to be to aid metamorphosis; the same substance more or less changed seems to be thrown out and re-absorbed until it be adapted for the repair of tissues, or become effete."

The reader will readily perceive how the system may become so charged that other organs of the body will vicariously attempt to play the part of a receptacle and conduit for the bowel, in order to excrete and eliminate ancient and offensive filth and bacterial poisons. The phenomenon of vicarious excretion may occur through the kidneys, lungs, skin, throat, nose, vagina, or uterus, thus keeping up chronic diseases and discharges that would not exist but for the chronic constipation or even for incomplete action of the bowels each day. Over-distention of the rectum, sigmoid and colon, due to the pressure of gases and the impaction of feces, results in inflammation, ulceration, stricture, appendicitis, abscess, strangulation, intussusception, and abnormal ballooning or roominess in certain portions of these intestines or conduits. This roominess, though it becomes filled with feces, and often with liquids, permits of sufficient space for even the daily passage of feces without dislodging the stored contents. The fact that there is a passage daily deceives both sufferer and medical adviser as to the source of the poisonous condition of the system, and masks the origin of such disorders as chronic inflammation and ulceration of the nose, throat, lungs, stomach, duodenum, colon, appendix vermiformis, uterus, bladder, kidneys and edema of the legs. But these evidences of auto-infection are generally preceded and accompanied by a general loss of vitality and weight, by anemia, by a lowering of the resisting power of the organism--all of which produce a fit soil for the various diseases to which flesh is heir. As soon as the system becomes saturated with bacteria and effete matter, auto-intoxication results, in which condition there is but little or no store of vitality for resistance, reaction and recuperation.

Dr. Bright has recorded several instances of fecal accumulation in the colon mistaken for enlargement of the liver and for malignant tumors. In one of the cases there was jaundice which disappeared after free evacuation of the bowels. Frerichs also relates a case where enlargement from fecal accumulation was at first ascribed to a pregnant uterus, and subsequently, on the supervention of deep jaundice, to an enlarged liver, but in which purgatives dispelled the patient's anxiety about a diseased liver and at the same time her hopes for a child.

Dr. N. Chapman, in his Clinical Lectures (p. 304), says:

"The feces sometimes accumulate in distinct indurated scybala or in enormous masses, solid and compact. Taunton, a surgeon of London, has a preparation of the colon and rectum of more than twenty inches in circumference containing three gallons of feces, taken from a woman, whose abdomen was as much distended as in the maturity of pregnancy. By Lemazurier, another case is reported of a pregnant woman, who was constipated for two months, from whom, after death, thirteen and one-half pounds of solid feces were taken away, though a short time before between two and three pounds had been scraped out of the rectum. Cases are reported by Dr. Graves of Dublin, which he saw in women, where from the great distentions in certain directions of the abdomen, the one was considered to be owing to a prodigious hypertrophy of the liver, and the other of the ovary; in the latter of which he removed a bucket-full of feces in two days. Mr. Wilmot of London has recently given a case where a gallon of matter was lodged in the cecum, and the intestines perforated by ulceration."

Dr. Pavy, in his treatise on The Functions of Digestion (p. 232), writes:

"The morbid conditions that constipation may occasion are of various kinds. Under an undue retention of fecal matters within the colon noxious products may be formed there, and act as irritants upon the mucous coat, setting up inflammation, followed by ulceration. It is to be here remarked that fecal matters are sometimes retained in the sacculi or pouches of the colon, and may give rise to the circumstances referred to, whilst a passage exists along the centre of the canal that shall permit a daily evacuation to occur. The dejections, even, may be loose in character, and still the same sequence of events ensue. From the irritating influence of preternaturally retained feces, colicky pains are, as a rule, induced, and the ultimate effects may be such as to lead to the production of fatal inflammation.

"The effect of constipation upon the muscular coat of the bowel is, through distention to which it is subjected, to weaken or deteriorate its evacuating power. As the result of a great amount of distention, like as happens in the case of the urinary bladder, more or less complete paralysis is induced. From the prolonged retention of fecal matter accompanying constipation, excrementitious products that ought to be eliminated become absorbed and thereby contaminate the contents of the circulatory system. As the result of this contamination, the secretions become vitiated, and a general disturbance of the conditions of life is produced. The action of the liver becoming deranged, its eliminative office is imperfectly discharged, and thus sallowness of the face and a bilious-tinged conjunctiva are produced. A coated tongue, foul mouth, loss of appetite, and other dyspeptic manifestations, accompany the general disorder of the digestive organs that prevails. The accumulation existing in the colon leads to a sense of distention and uneasiness in the abdomen. The kidneys vicariously discharge products that ought to have been eliminated by the alimentary canal. In this manner the urine becomes preternaturally loaded. From the contaminated state of the blood the functions of animal life also become disturbed; and hence the lassitude, debility, headache, giddiness and dejected spirits, that form such frequent accompaniments of constipation.... A distended cecum, colon, and rectum may also, by the pressure exerted upon the nerves and vessels of the lower extremities, be the cause of numbness, cramps, pains and edema of the legs. The edema occasioned by constipation, if not exclusively confined to one side, will in all probability be decidedly greater in one leg than in the other."

Case (from Gaz. Paris, July 20, 1839): A woman of fifty was troubled with habitual diarrhea and frequent calls to urinate, in which urine could be discharged only by drops. After six years of suffering and unsuccessful use of remedies, she was examined for the first time per anum, and an accumulation of fecal matter discovered, forming a mass the size of an infant's head. This was removed and found to weigh four pounds. She then got well.

CHAPTER VI.

HOW AUTO-INFECTION AFFECTS THE GASTRIC DIGESTION, AND VICE VERSA.

Frederick the Great said that all culture comes through the stomach. This saying emphasizes pithily the dependence of psychology upon physiology. The stomach with the intestines is certainly the source from which every portion of the body receives its nourishment and most of its diseases. The physiological plus and minus processes leave their reflex on the mind.

Prof. Ch. Bouchard, in his lectures on Auto-Intoxication (Oliver's trans., p.

14), says: "The organism in its normal, as in its pathological state, is a receptacle and a laboratory of poisons. Amongst these some are formed by the organism itself, others by microbes, which either are the guests, the normal inhabitants of the intestinal tube, or are parasites at second-hand, and disease producing."

In the preceding chapters we have mentioned some of the most common cases of retention of excreta in the rectum, sigmoid cavity, colon, cecum, duodenum and stomach, and how the consequent foul conditions often resulted in diarrhea. Auto-infection impairs the functions of every organ in the body, by clogging the pores with poisons and filth. By the transfer of disease germs from one infected, that is, tainted, contaminated part of the body to parts that were free from infection, the kidneys, mucous membrane and skin receive these unnatural products, and their functions are disturbed thereby. The disturbance of the various organs throughout the system sets up such a multiplicity of symptoms that one gets the impression of a pandemonium--a veritable council-hall of evil spirits. The visitation is omnipresent. Infliction, misery, are everywhere. The taint of auto-generated intestinal morbific products, carried and communicated to the remotest parts, manifests itself now here now there as if it were a local trouble, and it is difficult therefore, nay, impossible, to classify scientifically the symptoms of auto-infection. A classification, though necessarily imperfect, will aid in the diagnosis and treatment of the various abnormal conditions of the stomach and intestines, that is, of mal-digestion. The sympathy, good understanding and responsiveness between the brain and the digestive apparatus are so close and intimate that the physician must take into consideration the inter-relationship of these organs before deciding which one is reporting reflex nervous symptoms, and which direct symptoms. Plutarch says in one of his essays: "Should the body sue the mind before a court judicature for damages, it would be found that the mind had been a ruinous tenant to its landlord." The digestive apparatus is, or should be, a farm for the mind, but unfortunately it usually has to wait twenty or more years before the tenant understands how to cultivate it for the uses of his intellectual and esthetical life.

I have referred to the fact that the most common causes of constipation, indigestion and other foul conditions of the alimentary canal favorable to the production of autogenetic poisons and their auto-infection, are such common and every-day matters, so familiar to almost every one that the victim, the parents and the physician feel no alarm of the coming danger for years. During these ignorant and innocent years the poison and filth were being absorbed, infecting the system with their morbific taint and lowering the quality of the blood and lessening its quantity, producing the state known as anemia. Associated with progressive anemia is mal-assimilation, improper nutrition, ebbing of the nervous and vital forces and the lessening of the secretory, excretory and digestive powers. By the time the poor victim is weighing fifteen to twenty-five pounds less than he ought to the symptoms of ill-health are sufficiently alarming to compel the sufferer to seek medical aid for disease of the stomach, bowels, liver, kidneys, lungs, etc.

Slow digestion is perhaps the most common form of functional disturbance of the stomach, due to an insidious auto-infection for years. The eyes and the skin begin to show the effect of the poisonous infection. The skin becomes dry, pale and muddy in color; has more or less annoying eruptions, and exhibits a jaundiced appearance. The body is ill nourished, the nervous system depressed, the blood impoverished, the memory failing, the general appearance languid, irritable, anxious. What a household picture this is to every one of the human family! But let us fill it out somewhat more fully. Note how the undue delay of food in the stomach occasions a sense of weight and oppression, the feeling beginning about an hour after a meal and continuing for hours, sometimes attended with fermentation and sometimes without it. At times there is a feeling of drowsiness due to the absorption of an excessive amount of the gases which distend the stomach and bowels, and this absorption is accompanied by pains in the stomach, head, between the shoulders and in the region of the heart. Sleep is disturbed by dreams, or one is awakened with a feeling of numbness and palpitation of the heart. At times the urine is scanty, strongly acid or high-colored. The tongue is more or less foul, with white or creamy coating. Now and then tasteless or saltish eructations occur. The appetite may be too good, or there is no appetite at all. Note the careworn expression, the wondering what to eat, what to drink or what remedy to take. So between much worse and some better, the trouble continues--both of body and mind.

Indigestion, however, with undue formation of acids proper, or acids unnatural, to the stomach, is a much more annoying affliction than slow digestion. The sufferer from indigestion may be debilitated, anemic, may have a general want of tone; or he may be a more or less vigorous and plethoric person. In some cases flatulence is very troublesome. But the most usual symptoms are heartburn, acid eructations that produce burning sensations, sour taste at intervals or constantly in the mouth, setting the teeth on edge. In the more vigorous or plethoric sufferers a gouty diathesis may exist, which may result in a tendency to inflammation, bringing on neuralgia, rheumatism, gout, etc. Tongue more or less foul; uric acid in the system; confusion in the mind; headaches; pains in the loins, legs and feet; in fact, more or less shifting pains everywhere: these are the common exhibits of indigestion. On the whole, the sufferer is a victim to an irritable body and a fretful mind, necessitating the cultivation by him of patience and the effort to be agreeable.

Besides the symptoms mentioned, indigestion may also be accompanied by gastric pain or by uneasiness at the pit of the stomach. It may be a sense of fulness or tightness, or a feeling of distention or weight, or again, a feeling of emptiness, goneness or sinking. Now and then there are burning, tearing, gnawing, dragging sensations under the breast-bone; and there is a general complaint of a capricious appetite, heartburn, vomiting, nervous headache, neuralgia and cold extremities. Other symptoms are pain from lack of food at the proper hour, or from food taken at the improper time; both of which practices may be followed by flatulency, occasioning a swollen, drum-like condition of the stomach and abdomen; the body of the tongue will be coated white, while the edges will present a redder appearance than in health.

Impaired digestion with nervous symptoms--in which the morbid sensibility of the mind is apparently the greatest--is called hypochondria. This class of sufferers, whose bodily and mental ills and morbid fears are so chaotically interwoven, are deserving of much consideration. So numerous are their fears and so fertile are their reasons for the many changes they arbitrarily make in their efforts to get well or keep from getting worse, so obstinately sure are they of being always right--that we can but give them our sincerest pity.

In some cases the functional troubles of the stomach and mind are aggravated by disease of the pelvic organs, which adds to the depression of the mind through nervous sympathy with the abdominal organs.

Dr. Cullen says on this point:--

"In certain persons there is a state of mind distinguished by a concurrence of the following circumstances: a languor, a listlessness, or want of resolution and activity with respect to all undertakings; a disposition to seriousness, sadness and timidity as to all future events; an apprehension of the worst or most unhappy state of them; and therefore, often upon slight grounds, an apprehension of great evil. Such persons are particularly attentive to the state of their own health, to every smallest change of feeling in their bodies; and from any unusual feeling, perhaps of the slightest kind, they apprehend great danger and even death itself. In respect to all these feelings and apprehensions, there is commonly the most obstinate belief and persuasion." (Quoted in Leared, On Imperfect Digestion, p. 106.)

CHAPTER VII.

HOW AUTO-INFECTION AFFECTS INTESTINAL DIGESTION, AND VICE VERSA.

Intestinal indigestion is a more common form of functional disturbance than is gastric indigestion. It is a well established fact that the greater portion of the digestive work is done beyond the stomach, in the duodenum, by the hepatic and pancreatic fluids. The duodenum--very properly called the second stomach--has none of the peculiar characteristics of a receptacle that receives crude substances--the office of the stomach. Much greater sensitiveness characterizes the digestive canal than the stomach; which is accounted for by the fact that a network of nerves, forming the sympathetic system, surrounds the bowels. The symptoms of intestinal indigestion are not always clearly defined and distinguishable from gastric indigestion, especially as the two are frequently associated.

The cecum, more than any other portion of the digestive canal, resembles the stomach, and it secretes an acid, albuminous fluid having considerable solvent properties. It is to be observed that as the cecum is only three inches in length and two and a half in diameter, and as its contents are necessarily propelled in opposition to gravity, a slight casualty will hinder or obstruct the upward movement of the pultaceous mass of the effete ingesta. The turning point in the ascending colon affords another ready hindrance to the upward and onward movement of this mass; and the gases and ancient feces beyond the turn conduce to further sluggish peristalsis, bringing about more or less obstruction and reflex irritation of the remaining length of intestinal canal. Undue retention of the contents of the cecum, and the disturbance and obstruction of the duodenum by the pressure incident to the distention of the colon with feces and gases, lead to congestion, inflammation and occasionally to ulceration of the mucous membrane in various parts of the intestinal tube.

This condition of affairs increases the occlusion (closing) of the bowels, but makes very easy indeed the entrance and propagation of micro-organisms in the sub-mucous coat of the intestine. The conditions are now ripe and rife for auto-infection. Which of the following microbes are the most active agents of progressive auto-infection: the streptococcus lanceolatus, the bacterium pyogenes, the bacillus subtilis, the staphylococci, the bacterium coli commune? They all play a part in the game, reducing the body in time to a charnel-house. Or are such substances as putrescein, cadaverin, skatol or indol--which are derived through chemical change in the putrescent mass--

contributors to the spread of the poisonous taint throughout the system? Any single one or a group of the fifty or more bacterial poisons may be the responsible agents in the ensuing auto-infection. Chemical analysis of the gases resulting from decomposition reveals oxygen, nitrogen, hydrogen, carbonic acid, protocarbonated hydrogen and sulphureted hydrogen, ammonia, and sulphate of ammonia. Leucin, tyrosin, lithic acid, lithates, xanthin, cystin, keratin, sulphureted hydrogen, etc., are deposits in the urine and are signs of the derangement of the intestinal canal and liver. The external symptoms observed are the following: the tongue is large, pale, flabby and indented by the teeth at the edge of the anterior third, while its surface is white and the papill?often enlarged; the appetite may be excellent, though there is great functional derangement of the liver with lithemia, so that the sufferer is tempted to eat what he knows from experience will disagree with him; a bitter coppery taste in the mouth, due to taurocholic acid--a common symptom of lithemia or of imperfect oxidation of albumen; emaciation, fatigue, depression, headache, buzzing in the ears and deafness, disturbance of sight, loss of memory, faintness and vertigo, very marked in some cases; sometimes tenderness and pain under the cartilages of the right ribs; the fretting of the sensitive surface of the bowels by imperfectly digested, semi-putrescent food, resulting sometimes in convulsions, coma, paralysis, or in fetid diarrhea of an acid character producing a burning sensation or pain of the anus when the discharges are being passed; rumbling and twisting sensations in the region of the navel occurring with flatulency, and occasionally colicky pains which at times are so severe as to simulate poisoning.

In some people certain articles of food, without being either toxic or putrid, induce indigestion and the production of microbes in quantity amounting to one third of fecal dejections. Prof. Ch. Bouchard says:

"The consequence of this development of acid in the whole length of the digestive tube is an inflammatory condition. We notice catarrh of the stomach, ulcerative gastritis, to which patients often succumb after twenty-five years of bad stomach; these are the false cancers, as they are called, or malignant gastritis without tumor. The large intestine is inflamed; around the fecal matter are seen glairy secretions and sometimes blood (membranous enteritis)." (Op. cit., p. 159.)

In chronic inflammation of the rectum and colon there is more or less discharge of mucous, and in some cases of membranous, desquamation, with yellow or bloody mucus. The shreds, cords or complete tubular casts are discharged constantly or at varying intervals. The quantity and character often alarm the sufferer. The discharge is nothing less than a thick, tenacious mucus that had formed a thin coating on the inflamed mucous membrane, and become exfoliated in casts or thin shreds--the result of many years of morbid intestinal exaggerated action.

Microscopical examination of the desquamated intestinal membrane and mucus from a man forty years of age, revealed the following products: crystals, mostly complete; incomplete phosphates, very numerous; mucous shreds in abundance; fat globules and granules, numerous; anal epithelia; red blood globules, few; connective tissue, scanty; pus corpuscles, very few; margaric acid and detritus (substances resulting from the destruction or wearing away of the part); undigested material, mostly cellulose; leptothrix threads, micrococci; and the bacillus coli communis. Diagnosis: foul, undigested material, due to a chronic inflammation of the lower intestinal tract. The microscopical examination of mucus and desquamated membrane from a woman sixty-five years of age, disclosed that she was suffering from proctitis and colitis. She wrote: "Please tell me how long this mucous discharge must continue. I am alarmed at the quantity of membrane, cords, casts, etc., in my excreta, and I think that if this process goes on much longer there will soon be no bowels left to purify." This letter was written some weeks after contracting a severe cold, which accounts for the unusual amount of exfoliation and mucus. The sample she sent contained a large quantity of mucus, both threads and corpuscles; with a moderate number of epithelial scales, partly anal and partly intestinal. Pus corpuscles were present in small numbers; also vegetable fibres, fat, starch, muscle fibres and cellulose--the remains of undigested material. In the membranes themselves no micro-organisms were found; in the pieces containing undigested material the bacillus coli communis was found as well as micrococci, and the bacilli of putrefaction (secondary formation) were seen.

CHAPTER VIII.

THE CAUSE OF CONSTIPATION AND HOW WE IGNORANTLY TREAT IT.

One of the best preparations for active life is a first-class intestinal canal.

"An old Scotch physician," says Sir Astley Cooper, "for whom I had a great respect and whom I frequently met in consultation, used to say to me as we were about to enter our patient's room together, 'Weel, Misther Cooper, we ha' only twa things to keep in meend, and they'll serve us for here and herea'ter; one is au'ways to hae the fear o' the Laird before our e'es, that'll do for herea'ter; and th' t'other is to keep our boo'els au'ways open, and that'll do for here.'"

A person whose mind is devoted to the realization of ideals, and whose body has a set of bowels that perform the act of defecation twice every twenty-four hours is doubly prepared for a useful life.

"If thou well observe In what thou eat'st and drink'st, seek from thence Due nourishment, not gluttonous delight, Till many years over thy head return: So may'st thou live, till like ripe fruit thou drop Into thy mother's lap, or be with ease Gathered, not harshly plucked, for death mature."

Milton's advice in poetic lines is all very well for those who have escaped chronic inflammation of the lower bowels, an ailment common and troublesome even under the very best dietetic regulations.

Inflammation having once penetrated the circular and longitudinal muscular fibres or bands of a section of the intestine, all hope of a comfortable existence is at an end, for such inflammation will bring on constipation and constipation nervous misery. It is inevitable that inflammation should determine this outcome since it induces spasmodic contraction of the muscular walls of the tube, lessening the bore or closing the portion of the canal invaded. Plastic infiltration takes place in the walls of the gut, thickening and binding them together; or, if the inflammation be of a simple catarrhal or atrophic nature, the plastic infiltration will more or less bind the circular muscular bands of the gut together in their abnormally contracted state! The presence of feces and gases above the zone of the disease will increase the irritation and contraction of the affected portion of the intestine. Consequent upon these changes wrought by inflammation, gases and excrementitious material are perforce imprisoned in the intestine, inducing constipation, foul fermentation, flatulency, diarrhea, indigestion, nausea, loss of appetite, sick headache and, in fine, autogenetic poisons, the source of auto-infection, ending in auto-intoxication, the chronic poisoned condition of the system.

Since the most common cause of chronic constipation, internal sluggishness and uncleanliness, is known, too much cannot be said in condemnation of the wide-spread abuse of "liver and atony persuaders" and the use of irritating suppositories and dilating bougies, candles, etc. The numerous and various drastic purgative nostrums--which literally fill our medical literature--and the universal demand for them, are evidence of this very common disease, which disease is rendered worse by the drugs taken for the relief of a foul intestinal alveus. An abnormal amount of watery secretion is forced by the drug into the foul canal, to mix there with its contents, of which the major portion is retained and re-absorbed into the system. And to make the bad condition and treatment worse, all such sufferers, as a rule, drink very little water, some scarcely any.

The demand for an irritating stimulus to "open the bowels" (the exciters contribute to close them) is largely due to the popular error in thinking, "I can treat my own bowels quite as well as the doctor, if not better." No intelligent person would think of stimulating and irritating daily an inflamed region of tissue on the outer portion of the body; yet this is precisely what intelligent persons do when they habitually use liver and peristaltic persuaders. The primary disease in the lower bowels and the consequent symptoms are gradually aggravated as the "physic" habit is formed.

As in the case of opium fiends and drunkards, so with habitual cathartic drug-users, should they be suddenly deprived of the accustomed artificial stimulus and irritant they become absolutely miserable, mentally and physically. It is a well-known physiological fact that every artificial stimulation of the intestines is followed by a corresponding loss of vitality and reaction. Now that the almost universal cause of undue retention of foul, effete matter has been ascertained, it is important to communicate to the world at large the best means of cleansing the bowels without increasing the local primary disease and its annoying symptoms.

That external physical cleanliness is next to godliness is an apt proverb. That internal physical cleanliness is nearer to godliness no one will deny.

Water is a universal solvent and therapeutic agent and is therefore indispensable in the cleansing and purifying of the integument and mucous membrane of the body. A large quantity of water is necessary to carry on the functions of the animal economy. Water enters every cell and fibre of the living organism, aiding in nutrition and in the elimination of worn-out tissues which if retained turn into poisons.

It is really not an intelligent but rather a barbarous practice to prescribe liver and intestinal exciters for the purpose of throwing into the alimentary tract a sufficient quantity of watery excretions to "cleanse itself"; to succeed they must first soften and liquefy the dry, hardened feces and scybalous masses (little ancient, bullet-like formations) imprisoned above an inflamed and fevered lower bowel, even colon.

Normal feces consist of 75 per cent water; and when unduly retained in the colon much of this fetid percentage is absorbed into the system. Then drugs are prescribed to liquefy the hardened putrid remnant and absorption begins again: a fact very shocking to a sensitive, even sensible, person.

CHAPTER IX.

CURES FOR CONSTIPATION: "FEARFULLY AND WONDERFULLY MADE."

Diseases of the anus and rectum are very common, very numerous and of very critical consequences. This is especially true of the disease of chronic inflammation, one of whose symptoms is piles or hemorrhoids. In the writings of the early Greek and Roman physicians will be found minute descriptions of the latter disorder. But on the whole, the most important symptom of chronic inflammation of the lower bowel, and the most far-reaching in its morbific results, is that protean monster, chronic constipation. It deranges more lives, from infancy to old age, than any other pathological condition that can be named.

For the cause and cure of that mere symptom of a disease, constipation, the so-called scientific physicians, from the early history of medication to the present time, have had one immutable theory as to the leading cause, and one grand motto as to the "safe and sure" cure. They have always prescribed remedies for this malady on the theory of portal congestion and hepatic derangement, and hence their supreme motto: "Physic! Physic!! Physic!!!"

The layman naturally adopted the theory and the motto of his medical advisers; hence in his self-medication and also under advice he consumes such vast quantities of purgative nostrums.

I have just received some medical literature beginning with the usual salutation--"Dear Doctor"--setting forth a new and remarkable theory of the cause, and an original motto for the cure, of constipation. Its authors have discovered that the "rectal nerve-tissues" are hungry, torpid, anemic, and to overcome the "atony" they must be "Fed! Fed!! Fed!!!"

"The greatest of physical ills in America," we are informed, "is digestive torpor or semi-paralysis, originally induced by a kind of starvation of the intestinal nerve-tissues. One of its most prevalent forms is constipation," caused by "local torpor or semi-paralysis, dependent upon an anemic condition of the nerve-tissues of the rectal region." By "feeding directly" the limpid, bedraggled rectum and colon, they receive their "appropriate nutriment, by which comes added vigor,"--the nutriment the stomach and the rest of the system had failed to furnish on account of constipation, excessive fermentation, indigestion and auto-infection.

To overcome this "atony" of two or more feet of the lower bowel, a little "nutritious" suppository, weighing twenty grains, is a "specific." It is claimed to cure chronic auto-infection and the spasmodic occlusion of the lower bowel! The excessive activity of all the region invaded by the chronic inflammation and the local irritation are perpetuated by such "feeding" instead of allayed! Does it not stand to reason that there is already too much activity, and that when the irritability reaches a certain stage diarrhea or looseness of the bowels must result? Twenty grains prescribed once a day to nourish an organ (the rectum) six to eight inches in length, and from one and a half to two and a half inches in diameter! When for two to three feet the lower bowel requires nourishment, a suppository night and morning is prescribed! However, the new treatment has the merit of some consistency between the diagnosis and the treatment, notwithstanding both are wrong.

Chronic inflammation of the lower bowel causes, as I have pointed out, excessive activity and thereby excessive nutrition of the tissues involved in the morbid process. But sphincter ani gymnastics have been suggested by some one who thinks chronic constipation is owing to a lack of muscular activity of the lower bowels; and the following reason is given:

"Physiological experiments have shown that rapid voluntary movements of the external sphincter ani and the levator ani produce very active peristaltic movements of the large intestine. This effect is produced by the mechanical excitement of the plexus myentericus of Auerbach. This curious automatic center lies between the two muscular coats of the intestine and controls the peristaltic movements. A person suffering from constipation should make powerful movements of the sphincter ani, and of the levator ani, in as rapid succession as possible, continuing the exercise for three or four minutes or until the muscles are fatigued. The time chosen for this exercise should be either before breakfast or an hour after breakfast, according to the natural habit of the individual in respect to the evacuation of the large intestines."

There are surgeons who recommend stretching and paralyzing the external sphincter muscle; and if they are correct in their diagnosis and treatment, those who prescribe bile-bouncers, and those who prescribe "nutrient suppositories," and those who prescribe the use of rubber bougies and candles, should call a convention (to meet in, say, New York City) to discuss the subject and see if they cannot agree to inform the people that constipation is a sign of, or a factor in, the evolution of the human race. Those who believe in the gymnastics of man's ears and of his sphincter ani and the therapeutic merits of this and of that could readily assent to the same glorious conclusion.

Strange to say, there are in New York physicians who are in the habit of inserting a rubber bougie up their patients' rectums two or three times a week for the cure of constipation. Some, more bold, intrust the bougie performance to the patient in order that a daily dilatation and stimulation may be kept up until "recovery from the disease is effected." Others, more original, order the patient to insert a candle some six inches in length up the rectum and allow it to remain ten minutes, with the hope of a "rapid cure."

A Mrs. P----, who had used the candle treatment for a great length of time by order of her distinguished physician, once consulted me. On examination, I found her afflicted with atrophic catarrh, chronic constipation and anal ulceration, from which she had suffered for seven years, with but little intermission from pain during each day of that entire period.

CHAPTER X.

BILIOUSNESS AND BILIOUS ATTACKS.

Commonly the source of chronic gastro-intestinal uncleanliness, of dyspepsia, of autogenetic poisons and auto-infection is inflammatory occlusion--more or less permanent or spasmodic--of some part of the lower bowel. Many years of auto-infection will exhibit such diseased symptoms as poor appetite, bad digestion, impoverished blood, emaciation, etc., accompanied by increased virulence of the catarrhal discharge of mucus, shreds, etc., and a mind and body sinking down to the morbid plane of hysteria, hypochondriasis (fear of illness) and neurasthenia (debility of the nervous system).

Biliousness and bilious attacks are evidence that there is a more or less constipated condition, that there has been an occasional imprudence in diet, and that the dreadful sense of fulness up to the end of the tongue is a faithful report of the state of affairs. What is it but a full foul condition of the digestive canal, a complete blockade of the canal from the rectum or colon to the stomach, making the victim feel that there must be something done in the way of cleaning out? He fears that the condition will be followed by fever--not infrequently this is the case. Biliousness is usually supposed to be occasioned by hindrance to the flow of bile, and the conclusion is drawn that the liver requires stimulating. This supposition is erroneous and very far from pathological veritude, as the liver, like the other organs, is merely a secondary sufferer from the over-eating and the closed sewer.

"The bowels with sullen vapours cloud the brain, And bind the spirits in their heavy chain; Howe'er the cause fantastick may appear, The effect is real, and the pain severe."

The bilious attack is usually noticed in the morning before food has been taken. The tongue is heavily coated and often so foul that it is necessary to scrape it and cleanse the mouth of disagreeable taste. Eructations, nausea followed by vomiting of undigested foul-smelling food, and if the vomiting be long-continued, mucus from the stomach and bile that had accumulated in the duodenum, are sufficient evidence that there was no torpidity of the liver. There is likewise more or less headache, neuralgia, giddiness, hebetude (state of mild stupidity), dejection, confusion of the senses, skin disease, acne rosacea (scarlet redness of the nose and cheeks), eczema, etc. The headache may be seated in the centre of the brain and extend to one or both eyeballs and be increased by stooping. Should diarrhea occur many of the annoying symptoms are likely not to be present.

In this form of indigestion the bowels are often much constipated, which is usually only a more marked symptom of chronic constipation. The system now and then vigorously rebels against this chronic condition and an acute bilious attack is the evidence of such rebellion. The whole digestive canal is involved in the rebellion, resulting in the symptoms described and also in a morose, petulant and querulous temper, accompanied by a peculiar, despairing expression,--partly due, perhaps, to regrets of having only one digestive apparatus,--or in some cases, perhaps, of having any.

That the character and disposition may be materially influenced by such a state of the bowels is well established. Plato believed that "an infirm constitution is an obstacle to virtue, because such persons think of nothing but their own wretched carcasses"; for which reason he contended that Aculapius should not undertake to patch up persons habitually complaining, lest they beget children as useless as themselves, being persuaded that it was an injury both to the community and to the infirm person himself that he continue in the world, even though he were richer than Midas.

Acting on this well-known fact, the celebrated Voltaire, in one of the articles in his Philosophical Dictionary, has very humorously ascribed half the evils of Europe to the intestinal irritations of the public men of the age.

"Let the person," he adds, "who may wish to ask a favor of a minister, or a minister's secretary, or kept mistress, endeavor previously, by all means, to ascertain whether they go to stool regularly; and, if possible, to approach them after a comfortable evacuation, that being a most propitious moment, one of the mollia tempora fandi, when the individual is good-humored and pleased with all around him."

CHAPTER XI.

KING LIVER AND BILE-BOUNCERS.

The "house not made with hands"--the human body--has, like the house made with hands, its sewer system, which is over twenty-five feet in length. To cleanse (?) this wonderfully delicate, tortuous and extended passage-way of waste material, civilized man knows no better than to put in at the top of the house, purgatives, cathartics, bile-bouncers, etc., with one hope and purpose in view, namely, that these policemen go searching, scouring and hustling the intestines in the greatest possible haste, in order to remove an obstruction about three hundred inches distant from where these "forcers" had entered the intestinal sewer. With mercury as a scavenger the work is pretty thoroughly done, though extra care has to be taken that some of the teeth may remain after the victim survives the additional intestinal inflammation occasioned by its drastic measures.

Traits acquired by the father are inherited by the children; present-day doctors follow early practitioners; they still pour in many and various decoctions at the top of the obstructed sewer of the human house to dislodge accumulated gases and feces at the bottom. The plumber treats the sewer of the house of brick and stone more wisely.

Our fathers partook of laxatives, cathartics, purgatives, and in consequence we start in life with teeth, intestines, appendices, out of gear and nervous systems on edge. With unconscious stupidity we continue the fatuous practice. The monarch selected to preside over the functions of human life was the Liver; and it is only with bated breath that any doctor dares question the legitimacy of that monarch's claim. The loyal subjects of King Liver are ever ready to call out "quack," "charlatan," etc., to those who dare repudiate the sovereignty of the Liver.

So much attention and flirtation does the liver receive from the liver-persuaders that the pancreas ought to be very jealous. The pancreas excretes quite as much fluid into the duodenum as its larger neighbor, and is, therefore, no mean organ. And we need not wonder should we find the intestinal glands piqued at our over-attention to the liver, as they, in their work at the metamorphosis of digested food into blood, excrete two or three gallons of fluid in a day to the liver's two or three pints; yet witness our medieval solicitude for the liver, for one among many organs. The liver is located near the upper portion of the intestinal canal and connected by a tube (the bile duct) to the rest of the excursion route. The following liver-persuading knights-errant are prescribed and ordered by disciples of Hippocrates, Galen, Herodicus, and Iccus, to treat with that digestive and eliminative monarch, the Liver--usually at night-time, that the family may not be disturbed. After making as good terms as possible they journey on, riotously churning and swashing the long, tortuous canal and its contents in search of ancient toxic gases and feces lodged in the lower bowel. It is believed by the prescribers that the length of the journey adds dignity to the drastic, dredging knights-errant. The reader needs no introduction to the podophyllins, the aloes, the jalaps, the rhubarbs, the mercurys, the croton oils, the sennas, the salines, the seltzers, the Carters, the Beechams, the Websters, the Pierces, the Ayers, the Ripans, the Warners, and others belonging to "The Four Hundred" fashionable grenadiers, with their credentials and stamp!

After these knights-errant have paid their respects to King Liver, and ended their long, tortuous and eventful journey, they depart and leave behind them burning and painful abdominal and anal regrets, and then some soothing, stimulating and tonic remedies are in order, so that the dredged though chronically constipated sufferer and his friends may still hope that life will be spared to repeat the same nauseating and often painful process in a few days or weeks, taking, in the meanwhile, milder bile-bouncers daily as a reminder to King Liver that the time for the knights-errant is coming again.

Sufferers from chronic constipation receive assurances that by the use of these "remedies" the anemia will be corrected, nutrition and digestion restored, atony of the liver and intestines overcome, yellow complexion and morbid feeling disappear. In short, remove the numerous symptoms and "causes" of toxicity of the body and of chronic constipation, and proclaim the victory of Powder and Pill!

All of us would believe Medicus, the son who so abjectly follows in the footsteps of his father, if we could really feel the possibility of such a victory; but the protests of our bowels are living witnesses against the validity of the medieval practice as here described; and we ask for a modern scientific solution of the fulness and foulness within and the fatuity without.

I must now apologize to the large class of sufferers from chronic constipation for hurting their feelings. I know very well how seriously they have been compelled to regard their trouble, and out of respect for their protracted suffering and efforts to get relief I should instead have sympathized and condoled with them in their dire misfortune. But we all know and realize that there are occasions when we get into awful and painful predicaments, and, when the whole situation is taken in, it becomes comical and ridiculous, so that for a time we cannot treat it seriously, even when old Chronic Biliousness and the mighty knights-errant are having a deadly combat at our internal and external (and possibly infernal) expense.

CHAPTER XII.

SEMI-CONSTIPATION AND ITS DANGERS.

"At least six times in every fleeting day Some tribute to the renal functions pay, And twice or thrice all alvine calls obey."

What has been said thus far has been based on chronic constipation mainly, and the accompanying intestinal foulness, which condition was shown to be so annoying that it compelled the sufferer to resort frequently to some more or less direct and artificial means for the relief of the bowels and the incidental indigestion. It has been further shown that many of the chronic cases fail to take on the normal amount of flesh or lose what flesh they have because of self-poisoning (auto-infection), which in turn is the outcome of mal-assimilation and mal-nutrition, and that this consequence must occur wherever there is an absorption of waste through a checking or disturbance of systemic functions. Emaciation and anemia are inevitable in such cases. On the other hand, there are cases that have such great powers of assimilation and elimination that they are able to stand the invasion of destructive material, may maintain the normal amount of flesh, or even take on an abnormal amount, but with the invariable accompaniment of more or less impoverishment of blood, disturbed circulation, indigestion, and the usual nervous derangements. The harmful practice of the lean and the fleshy sufferers of resorting to daily medicines--cathartics, digestives and tonics--has been commented upon. Willingly do they squander their money to get relief from an ever-present ailment. Cases are these of hope deferred that maketh the heart sick.

The primary cause of chronic constipation, namely, proctitis, has been explained, and its many symptoms, as indicated by the functional disturbances of many or all of the organs of the body, enumerated.

But beside the cases of chronic constipation--both lean and fat--there are many sufferers from auto-infection who have only semi-constipation, or partial evacuation of the feces daily. Though they suffer from the effects of self-poisoning, yet they have no such well-defined symptoms of local disease and functional disturbance as are always found in those who have chronic constipation. Nevertheless, they have disturbances of practically all the functions of the system. Believing as they do that the evacuation of their bowels is complete, they are at a loss to find a cause for the toxemia (blood-poisoning), mal-nutrition, debility and general atony. The symptoms of auto-infection with the semi-constipated are as complex as with the severer cases, but not so well defined. The most prominent symptoms are those connected with the process of katabolism, that is, of degeneration of the tissues, as indicated by their color and texture. The liver, however, is usually held responsible for the bad complexion, impaired nutrition, constipation and diminished vitality, when really the liver is only indirectly concerned, as made manifest in the previous articles. The seat and source are found to be the diseased colon and rectum.

Dr. Treves says: "The colon being the part of the bowel involved in obstruction due to fecal accumulation, it may be further assumed that the blocking of the gut will most usually concern its lower or terminal parts. Accumulation of feces is most common in the rectum and sigmoid flexure, and then in the cecum. Masses of feces may block the colon at any point, and more particularly at the flexures of the bowel. Still, the three common sites of the accumulation are those just named. The accumulation in the colon may assume the form of a more or less isolated nodule or mass. Thus a considerable lump may be found in the cecum or sigmoid flexure and the rest of the colon be comparatively clear of any gross accumulation. An isolated lump may even persist after free purgation. On the other hand, the accumulation may assume the form of several isolated fecal masses. One of them may occupy the cecum, another the transverse colon, and possibly a third the sigmoid flexure. The bowel between these masses may appear to be fairly clear."

A number of the exciting causes of inflammation of the lower or terminal portion of the large intestine have been mentioned. It cannot, however, be too strongly emphasized that chronic inflammation of the colon and rectum results in hyperkinesis (excessive muscular irritability) and contraction of the diseased portion invaded, thereby retarding or preventing the passage of feces and gases. A portion of the daily accumulation of feces in the sigmoid may pass through the diseased rectum every day, but not without increasing the inflammation and the spasmodic contraction; this in time inhibits the elimination of the accumulating feces, which by undue retention become condensed and hardened. Each day will then be a repetition of the abnormal and partial effort of the organ to accomplish the act of defecation, and there will be no thought of the cumulative and chronic intoxication (poisoning) of the system from the imprisoned feces and gases.

It may be stated without reservation that the rectal canal cannot be involved in chronic inflammation without involving the anal canal, and vice versa. One half of civilized people are suffering from chronic constipation, and very nearly the remainder from semi-constipation. The semi-constipated are now under consideration. The chronic cases are those that have a complete impaction of feces in the terminal portion of the sigmoid and rectum; the semi-constipated have the usual daily partial impaction, that is, an incomplete or partially successful evacuation of the contents of the bowels: the incompleteness is due to disease of the anal and rectal canals.

The anal and rectal canals are made up of circular and longitudinal muscular bands, which, when invaded by disease, lose their proper or normal sensibility and cooperative voluntary action. The excessive contraction of the circular muscles closes the calibre or bore of the gut, and the excessive contraction of the longitudinal muscles shortens the length of the gut, thus throwing the mucous membrane into abnormal folds which increase the depth of the sacculi, or cavities, between the fibrous folds. In the normal gut the sacculi and bands act as valves to control the descent of the feces. This valvular arrangement and the curvatures of the lower bowels conserve the energy of the involuntary and voluntary nerve force until there is a sufficient accumulation of feces to excite a normal desire for stool; otherwise the feces would rush upon the anus at once and occasion much inconvenience.

Catarrhal inflammation of the mucous membrane of the anal canal will sooner or later penetrate the muscular structure of that canal, causing an abnormal irritability and contraction of the sphincter ani and the other tissues composing its structure. The contraction of the anal tissues becomes more permanent as the muscular tissues of the structure become cohered or bound together by the process of inflammation.

The normal stimulus and sensation that should precede the act of defecation are perverted or destroyed by the excessively irritable contraction of the sphincter ani, which contraction is occasioned by the presence of feces and gases just above the seat of inflammation, that is, above the anal canal or at the lower end of the rectum. As the bulk of feces and gases lodged at this point increases, the anal contraction becomes firmer in grip, and as a consequence permits no hint of the imprisoned contents until the accumulating bulk is beyond the power of toleration by the organ. Daily a portion of the lodged feces, or some new addition to the mass, passes the anal canal, but the attending irritation or contraction of the muscles prevents any further exit of the imprisoned rectal contents.

CHAPTER XIII.

THE ETIOLOGY OF THE MOST COMMON FORM OF DIARRHEA, i.e., EXCESSIVE INTESTINAL PERISTALSIS.

If you are interested to know why a certain plant does not flourish in the temperature and light to which it has been accustomed, you investigate the soil--the source of nourishment--and thus determine why the downy or velvety appearance has left the flower; why the leaves are yellow, dry or falling; why the stems are withering. Even the most ignorant person knows that the symptoms the plant presents did not bring about the unsuitableness of the soil; that, on the contrary, the condition of the soil is responsible for the plant's present state. Would it not be unwisdom, therefore, to treat directly the symptoms of decay, instead of treating the soil, or changing it? Just so misguided is the judgment of the physician who prescribes physic or tonics in the case of a person having a foul intestinal canal, a condition destructive of the absorbent and the excretory glands. But members of county medical societies do just such foolish things. Notwithstanding their prescriptions, a point will be reached by the patient where the restoration of his millions of small rootlets, or organic feeders, will be impossible, and like a decaying plant in unfavorable soil he gradually decays or withers, here and there, until finally he topples over before he knows it, probably long before maturity has been reached.

It is not generally known among laymen, nor sufficiently appreciated among physicians, that the mass of fecal matter normally evacuated from the bowels comes mainly from the blood; and that this mass is not, as it is usually supposed to be, the residue of the food that has been left unassimilated. Embedded in the mucous membrane of the colon are tubular glands under the control of the nervous system. When these glands become unduly excited through local inflammation and irritation, the normal flow from them is increased to such an extent that a rapid waste of precious tissue occurs throughout the system, and the vital force--which had taken perhaps years to store--is depleted to the point of exhaustion, sometimes even in a few hours. Almost every one has had some experience of exhaustion following diarrhea.

The increased flow of blood to the mucous membrane of the colon furthers this extraordinary secretion by the glands. As has been pointed out, inflammation, septic poisoning, intestinal foulness, or retained feces, act as irritants on the mucous membranes, thereby drawing the blood to the colon where it is excreted and exhaustion follows. The great danger in diarrhea, therefore, is the rapid depletion of the vital force. But when the small intestines are affected the consequences may be still more deplorable. Then the unassimilated food is hurried along too quickly for absorption and the body receives but little nourishment to restore its powers. Thus another draught is made upon the sufferer's reservoir of vitality, and hence additional exhaustion. But this waste of tissue, loss of vital force, non-assimilation and non-supply, are not so grave as the positive danger of the permanent destruction of the millions of small absorbing vessels (villi) of the small intestine by a continuance of this abnormal irritation. Of course the secretory and excretory glands of the colon also suffer, and we then have costiveness resulting from lack of absorption and excretion.

Abnormal irritability of the bowels is necessarily involved in the inflammatory process known as proctitis and colitis. Increase this irritability to a certain point and diarrhea takes the place of constipation--a much more alarming symptom. Diarrhea is more alarming because the intensified local activity of the excretory glands of the bowels brings on, as has been said, a general exhaustion of the vital powers.

The severity of diarrheal symptoms is much increased by the character and abundance of bacterial poisons. Bacteria find a ready medium in fetid feces, and are absorbed by the excited glands to the degree in which these glands have time and power for absorption. Of course the extent and character of the intestinal irritation have a good deal to do with the severity of the diarrheal symptoms. This irritation is not infrequently intensified by a catarrhal process, or by a lesion of an ulcerative nature. All these forms of irritation bring on "excessive intestinal peristalsis"--which, accordingly, is our definition of diarrhea. The normal peristaltic action of the intestines propels the nutritive as well as the effete material through the canal at a rate that allows of both proper absorption and timely elimination. But when excessive peristalsis occurs, neither absorption nor elimination will be normal or suited to the requirements of the system.

Undigested foodstuffs may become an irritant, or increase, as is usually the case, the established irritation, and thus bring on an acute attack of diarrhea. The immediate consequence of the acute attack may indeed be, and often is, comparatively beneficial, inasmuch as the diarrhea removes the undigested material that occasioned the irritation. When this removal is accomplished, the diarrhea usually subsides without treatment. This is the case, however, only when the patient has committed an infrequent error in diet. When such errors are habitual the burden on the glands of the intestinal mucous membrane becomes intolerable, and the chronic inflammation once established has a tendency to proceed from bad to worse. It will then be observed that digestion becomes more and more impaired. In such a case diarrhea will no longer serve a good end, but will on the contrary debilitate the system. A change to better dietetic habits will then aid, but will not suffice for cure. Only treatment and time will restore the inflamed parts to a healthy tone. When, however, the digestive tract is invaded by any of the many forms of bacteria, treatment will avail little and serious consequences follow rapidly.

Too much cannot be said or done to secure intestinal cleanliness in infancy, childhood and maturity. Mothers and nurses cannot give this subject too much thought and care, since the welfare of future generations depends largely upon intestinal cleanliness, in view of the rich and racy life of our hothouse civilization. We are a people poisoned through constipation and diarrhea: two affections that derange more lives than all other pathological conditions together. Banish alimentary uncleanliness and you take most of the poisons from the human race--poisons that stunt the body and blunt the mind.

The soul of man should dwell in a palace, not in a pest-house; in a human temple, velvety, lined with down, inside and out; in which there are hundreds of millions of lilliputian trappings, fittings and articles of furniture, to carry on the minute and finer functions and chemistry of the soul. The very multitude of the fine equipments that decorate the temple give it that beautiful blending of color and form which its coating has when in normal condition. They adorn this body-house with health, and supply it with the rich red wine of joy.

The blood is dependent for its richness not only on the digestive fluids, but also on the proper eliminating powers of the system. If you would avoid premature decay you must not neglect the reservoir of vitality, the alimentary canal, but see to it that it be kept clean and pure. Then will the elixir of life spring from an almost inexhaustible fountain. To recur to our plant analogy. Keep the soil in your own vegetable garden sweet, for intestinal cleanliness corresponds to soil fitness. Purity of the stomach and bowels is more important than quantity or quality of food. That defecation should occur normally two or three times in twenty-four hours is more important than that three meals should be eaten within that time. The conveniences for eating and drinking are on every hand, but oh, how few, inaccessible, miserably constructed, and poorly cared for, are the toilet cabinets for the accommodation of the gourmand! Suspenders and silk hats mark the progress of our outer refinement; toilet cabinets and flushing appliances, of our inner. When the inner refinement comes we shall live longer and be healthier.

CHAPTER XIV.

BALLOONING OF THE RECTUM.

To make plainer what has been said of the rectal and anal tubes or canals, consider the sleeve of an infant's gown. This sleeve well represents the rectal tube, the wrist-band the anal orifice and tube--an inch or more long. Think of the sleeve or rectal tube as being made up of four layers of material or membranes; and counting from the inside of the sleeve or rectum there are (1) the mucous layer; (2) the areolar layer; (3) the muscular layer; (4) the serous layer.

The muscular membrane is itself composed of two layers, and may be said to form the framework of the rectum. One layer is composed of circular muscular fibres, and the other of longitudinal muscular fibres. In a similar manner you could make a sleeve out of fine circular rubber bands; then bind them together by rubber strings extending lengthwise of the sleeve. With the circular bands the bore of the sleeve may be contracted or widened; and with the longitudinal bands the length may be shortened or extended. Just so with the corresponding muscular membranes of the rectum, in their normal and abnormal conditions. Outside of the longitudinal muscular bands are the serous and areolar layers, the latter covering the lower half of the rectum.

As you look inside the incomplete model of the rectum, or rather sleeve, you observe circular muscular bands or fibres which it is necessary to cover with soft spongy or fatty substance in whose meshes are nerves, blood-vessels, etc. This is called the areolar layer or coat. One more layer or coat upon this--the mucous coat--completes the structure. This latter possesses the power of accommodating itself to the distention and contraction of the muscular tube. The mucous membrane is thrown into folds and columns which serve as valves to inhibit the undue descent of the feces, thus assisting the mucous membrane in performing its office.

The length of the rectum varies in different persons, six inches is the average length. It is divided into two parts. The upper part is a little more than three inches long; beginning in front of the third sacral vertebra and extending down to the end or tip of the coccyx. In shape this part conforms to the curve of the sacrum and the coccyx, to which it is attached behind. The lower part of the rectum is a little shorter than the upper part, and begins at the tip of the coccyx and extends down with the same curve as the upper part, terminating at the upper portion of the anal canal.

Returning to the sleeve again; the portion of it from the shoulder to the elbow illustrates the upper part of the rectum when partially covered with a serous coat on the side opposite the bore (the outside). From the elbow to the wrist-band illustrates the lower part of the rectum, when covered on the outside with an areolar coat.

The wrist-band of the sleeve will represent the anal tube if drawn into a pucker and turned slightly backward from the direction of the sleeve of which it is a continuation.

The muscular fibres described above likewise enter into the formation of the anal canal or orifice. This orifice is closed by two strong muscles that lie close together and are called internal and external sphincters, which are abundantly supplied with nerves and blood-vessels whose branches extend to the neighboring organs.

Nine persons in every ten have more or less chronic inflammation of the mucous membrane of the anus and rectum. In time the areolar and muscular coats become invaded by the morbid process, and this increases the irritability of the tissues of the organ.

The change from the normal functions of the anal membranes is slow, and the symptoms are not well marked and are consequently ignored for years owing to inexpertness in detecting an invading serious disease, until the time comes when the suffering can no longer be tolerated by the victim of the neglect.

The result of disease to muscular tissue is contraction of its fibres, and the contractions become more painful as the disease increases. Accompanying the inflammation, there is a more or less inflammatory product secreted between muscular fibres that "glues" them together in their contracted state. And as the anal and rectal tubes are made up of round muscular fibres, it is not hard to see how the bore of the canal can be lessened by the slow binding together of its fibres in the contracted state. The fact is that when the anal structure is invaded by inflammation, there is more or less stricture of the canal and of the orifice.

Recalling the sleeve illustration, and how the wrist-band was puckered and bent back a trifle so that the contents of the sleeve would not pass out so easily, suppose you now pucker the wrist-band rather tightly, and suppose there is a forcible descent of sand in the sleeve, the natural result would be a bulging out of the lower portion of the sleeve just above the wrist-band, or place of undue constriction. If the abnormally constricted condition of the anal orifice has been growing from bad to worse for years, the locality immediately above the anal canal will become dilated or cavernous (caused by retained feces or gases), which cavity is called ballooning of the rectum. When a speculum is introduced into the rectum (as shown on page 14 of pamphlet How to Become Strong), and through it a bent probe is inserted to determine the depth of the dilatation or abnormal cavity, it is as if one were poking inside of an inflated balloon: hence the name.

Anatomists describe the rectum as terminating in a forward pouch, which is close to the prostate gland in the male and the lower part of the vagina in the female. In some cases there may be such a slight pouch, due to the anal canal not following the direction of the rectum, and slightly turning backward; but in most cases such a normal pouch is not perceptible or observed through the speculum. The small pouch sometimes found on the anterior wall of the rectum I have thought due to a very acute inflammation on the verge of forming abscess, which often occurs in the triangular space. (See 4 in diagram in pamphlet cited above.)

Immediately above the sphincter muscles on the posterior wall of the rectum the greatest dilatation is found (as shown by the bent probe), and extends on each side with less depth about the anterior wall of the rectum.

The greater portion of the lower part of the rectum, which part is about three inches long, is usually involved in the dilatation or ballooning. Often the upper half or more of the anal canal is also dilated with the rectum, leaving the sphincter muscles quite bare of fatty tissue, with anal length of a quarter of an inch or less.

Your attention was called to a sleeve containing sand, and the bulging or dilatation above the puckered wrist-band that was an inch or more broad. Now suppose there were two strong rubber rings at the lower end of the wrist-band, whose power of resistance to pressure is much greater than the tissues above them forming the wrist-band. Naturally, the tissues which form the upper part of the wrist-band would dilate the same as the terminal portion of the sleeve just above the wrist-band.

Similar changes in structure or formation take place in diseases of the anal and rectal canals which result in ballooning of the rectum; and two frail constricted sphincter muscles are left to guard this balloon, filled, as it so often is, with feces and gas.

Chronic inflammation, that results in contraction of the circular muscular fibres, will sooner or later constrict the gut so that it will lose its normal power to expand without causing pain. The anal canal may be said to be strictured to the degree in which it is unable to dilate normally, and this strictured condition usually grows from bad to worse.

The first symptom of rectal disease is usually an affection of the anus, which affection occasions an inhibition, that is, a reluctant permission for the passage of the feces; and this inhibition results, consequently, in some degree of constipation. And this constipation reacts more or less on the peristaltic action of the bowels and in time defeats the function of peristalsis. All this will react on the inflammatory processes at the anus, which originally engendered the constipation. The narrow and contracted strait or canal through which the feces must pass, gives a tape-like shape to the stools.

The anal and rectal mucous membrane is of a firm and tough structure, similar to the integument at the bottom of a boy's heel. After many years' observation of diseases of the anus and rectum I am forced to conclude that as a rule inflammation exists in the tissues twenty or more years before the severe symptoms, such as piles, fissure, anal pockets, pruritus, hypertrophy, atrophy, tabs, abscesses, and fistula, are sufficiently annoying to compel the sufferer to seek medical aid. I believe it to be of as much importance to give early attention to disease of the anus and rectum as to teeth and eyes, or even more.

CHAPTER XV.

BALLOONING OF THE RECTUM--Continued.

In the last chapter a description was given of the anatomy of the anus and rectum; and it was shown how a chronic inflammatory process involving these organs develops stricture in the parts invaded; and it was shown how a partial stricture of the anal canal results in ballooning or dilatation of the lower part of the rectum. The primary cause of all the symptoms of rectal disease is chronic inflammation (proctitis) involving the whole structure of the anal tubes and in a few cases the sigmoid flexure as well.

Perhaps the first marked symptom of disease of the rectum is constipation, semi-constipation or of chronic character. The function of the anus and rectum being disturbed by the inflammation, the fecal mass is unduly retained and its moisture is absorbed by the system. This accounts for the condensed and hardened fecal mass in isolated lumps of various proportions.

A hard-formed stool is abnormal, and is evidence of auto-infection. When three-fourths of the normal fecal mass has been re-absorbed by the system, does it not stand to reason that the blood and tissues have been poisoned by their own waste products (auto-intoxication) and that anemia, emaciation and local disturbances of other organs of the body are symptoms of such intoxication?

The loading and blocking of the sigmoid flexure come from too much activity or irritability, due to inflammation, of the upper half of the rectal tube. A consequence of this excessive sensitiveness is a diminished or perverted normal stimulus, notice or desire, that the act of defecation should take place.

The victim of proctitis simply forms a habit of daily soliciting an evacuation, though the normal invitation or desire to stool may be entirely absent, and the evacuation in such cases is attended with more or less delay and straining effort to accomplish partially or wholly the expulsion of the more or less inspissated feces.

As the extreme sensitiveness of the inflamed upper half of the rectum offers resistance to the passage of the fecal contents of the sigmoid flexure; so, in a somewhat similar manner, the inflamed anal tube, in its more or less constricted state, prevents the passage of feces and gases as they approach the terminal part of the rectum. As a consequence, the feces and gas deposit and lodge at this latter location, producing in so doing the abnormal cavity called ballooning of the rectum, so often found just above the anal tube.

The greatest depth of the dilated pouch is on the posterior wall of the rectum, or just in front of the tip of the coccyx. In some cases the pouch measures two and a half inches in depth at the back and gradually diminishes in depth on each side as you near the anterior wall of the rectum. Often the upper end of the anal canal is higher than the depressed circumference of the spacious cavity that almost surrounds it. The irritable orifice of the cavity will invariably compel a quantity of liquids and feces to lodge in the cavity as a permanent cesspool, allowing the absorbent vessels to absorb as much as they can by incessant work. The height or length of this abnormal cone-shaped rectal cavity is from two to three inches, involving usually the lower half of the rectum. The anal canal frequently becomes shortened by the dilating process to a quarter of an inch, leaving two frail, irritable muscles at the vent, to guard the rectal cavity. And fortunate are these two thin, sore, contracted muscles, and the possessor of them, if they escape the surgeon's barbarous notion of operating on them.

If the medical butcher has operated on them, you will find an anal canal open to such an extent that two fingers can be inserted without distending the tissues in the least. And when the victim of ballooning of the rectum and ignorant operation makes further complaint to the surgeon of the aches and pains, he is consoled by being informed that the end of the spine will have to be removed. Irreparable damage done and no aid at all received! It is a pity such ignorance on the subject should exist in the medical profession in this city.

The abnormal cavity, so difficult to empty properly owing to its depth and diseased outlet, is seldom free from gases, feces and liquids. Daily evacuations will not empty this cavity, nor will cathartics or diarrhea. A permanent cesspool of poisons is this, where all forms of poisonous germs are propagated, and infect the system by absorption. No use to take medicines for your poor blood, bad complexion and horrid feelings, as they will not cleanse the augean stable so long neglected. No use to journey to other localities for health so long as you carry so formidable a foe to health with you.

The mucous membrane in the chronic state of the disease presents a rather dry, indolent and bluish appearance, except that here and there the tissues show more activity of the disease, more especially so over the anal region, due to harsher disturbance during the act of stooling. In the subacute or acute stage of the inflammatory process there is more general redness and puffiness of the mucous membrane, or a swollen condition with increased discharge of mucus and perhaps some blood.

There is a heavy, uncomfortable feeling, with more or less soreness and pain, especially after evacuation of the feces. If a fissure or anal ulcer is present the pain is in proportion to its size and the general aggravation of all the diseased parts. Itching or pruritus about the anus may accompany the trouble to a very annoying extent, being an evidence that the anal pockets are becoming much diseased. The partially constricted and irritable sphincter muscles become excited during the act of stooling and react on the anal grip or contraction, making it more intense. This latter condition may shut off the flow of blood in a local vein; and the blood becoming coagulated forms a painful bluish grape-like tumor at the external opening of the anus.

Abscesses may form at some portion of the diseased gut and result in an external fistula.

Piles may co-exist in some cases of ballooning, but are usually not annoying.

It is the local anal or external annoyances that compel the sufferer to seek medical advice and aid, and he learns that the troubles complained of are only symptoms of a chronic disease, therefore easily removed without harsh treatment while the cause is being properly cured.

It is very fortunate for the sufferer from ballooning of the rectum to have in or near the anal canal those painful hints or symptoms of a very grave and long existing disease whose constitutional symptoms were well marked but attributed to other causes, especially to disease of the liver--an organ of so much solicitude that the poor liver-worshipping patient ought to receive more gracious response from it.

In every case of chronic proctitis, or inflammation of the anus and rectum, the sigmoid flexure must be more or less dilated, as the upper part of the rectum is very irritable and contracted and inhibits the feces from passing beyond the sigmoid; but this irritability and contraction of the rectum, as a rule, is not nearly so severe as that of the anal canal, whose orifice is closed by very strong sphincter muscles.

Such being the pathological change in the sigmoid flexure and especially in the lower portion of the rectum, as described in these two chapters, who, with ordinary intelligence and an idea of cleanliness, would take or prescribe remedies to move the bowels, if it were possible to cleanse the foul capacious cavities with water? We know that they can be thus cleansed, and that it can be easily accomplished with benefit to the diseased canals.

After the system has absorbed 75 per cent of the fecal mass, a "remedy" is taken to excite a flow of watery excretions into the bowels, of which a portion will be retained in the colon, and especially the ballooned cavities, and reabsorbed; and every day the objectionable practice is repeated without any thought of the harm being done.

The flushing of the rectum, sigmoid flexure and colon with water is not a cure-all, but it is one of the means of treating a grave chronic disease, a disease insidious and far-reaching in its poisonous effects on the human organism.

CHAPTER XVI.

THE USUAL DIAGNOSIS AND TREATMENT OF BOWEL TROUBLES WRONG.

Herodotus tells us that among certain tribes when a man fell sick his next-door neighbor did not wait for him to become thin but killed him at once, lest by the loss of his adipose his flesh might be rendered less appetizing.

But alas! in this age of constipation and piles, of self-generated poisons and self-infection, how changed is the custom! Our next-door neighbor, the doctor, waits till we are really thin, and then begins to feed and grow fat on our ills! In our day, through the continuous process of self-poisoning we take on no flesh from puny, peaked childhood, or we insidiously lose what little flesh we had, and when our bones are well exposed, become alarmed, realize that we are sick, rush for the doctor, and dispossess ourselves of our spare cash.

Very frequently, as stated in the first chapter, auto-infection begins in infancy and slowly but steadily progresses, but it may not be before adult age is reached and one or more organs are seriously diseased that it becomes apparent to all. The vital round of the alternate building-up and breaking-down of the system has been going on unceasingly during these years of increasing infection, but prematurely the balance between up and down is lost in favor of down; the building-up process becoming feebler, slower, and the breaking-down process quicker, easier. What can the inevitable outcome be but emaciation and anemia, and all their attendant suffering and consequences? It is the superabundance of vitality in the growing child that retards (inhibits) the morbid changes going on in the blood and tissues of the system; but the process is all the more insidious by being thus restrained, and its very subtlety and stealth beguile us all into fancied security: parents, friends, physicians--all are deceived.

As stated in a previous chapter, the first unwelcome visitor, in infancy, is inflammation of the integument and mucous membrane of the anal orifice, invited by the uncleanliness involved in the use of diapers; and this visitor takes up its residence slowly along several inches of the lower bowel. Its first symptoms are likely to be constipation, flatulency, colic, indigestion, bacterial and other poisons, occasionally diarrhea, and the usual general disturbance of the system as above detailed. It is admitted by all authors that inflammation of the anus, rectum, etc., is by far the most common disease that afflicts mankind at all ages; and I maintain that the natural result of such inflammation is a more or less extensive occlusion of the lower bowel, which in turn involves an undue retention of the feces, and thus we have the foul intestinal canal and stomach called gastric and intestinal indigestion.

The wrong treatment of constipation, diarrhea, indigestion and auto-intoxication up to the present time has been due to improper diagnosis. Writers on these subjects speak of them as causes when they are merely symptoms. And the remedies for these "causes" are even more numerous. Mistaken diagnosis on the one hand, measured doses on the other, and there you have the scientific doctor! The primary cause, inflammation, like the original spark applied to dry shavings, sets up morbid changes in the various parts of the digestive canal and the other organs of the body, and these "set up" or established changes are properly secondary or derivative causes accompanied by their own symptoms. The primary disease and symptoms may exist for five, ten, twenty or more years before any pronounced secondary or derivative diseases and their symptoms occur or are noticeable to a sufficiently marked degree.

The chronic character of the malady, and the complication of primary with secondary diseases and their symptoms, have thoroughly disconcerted the doctors. Hence the many "causes" assigned for indigestion, constipation, etc., and the many kinds of remedies prescribed with the one sure result, FAILURE; and hence, also, not a few of the self- and drug-intoxicated ones dubbed, or actually developed into, hypochondriacs. Diagnosis wrong, treatment wrong, failure certain, and the foulness of the intestinal canal continued! This is the experience and testimony of the many, many sufferers from the most common malady that afflicts humanity from infancy to old age, and which will continue to afflict the great majority until it is properly understood and treated.

When a sewer of a town is obstructed, the most sensible plan is to begin the investigation at the outlet and then proceed up, section after section, to trace the obstacle that had occasioned the accumulation of debris. When the waste-pipes of a house are clogged, we do not expect the plumber to go to the top of the building and poke substances down the pipe to dislodge the unduly retained material some twenty-five feet or more away. Nor would we believe him if he informed us that the sewer-gas and overflow of waste in the house were the cause of the constipated condition of the drain. But just this is what the doctor declares concerning our sewer; just this is what he does when he doses it with laxatives, cathartics, purgatives. Such is the treatment we receive when we rush to the doctor, or such the treatment we give ourselves. The poor, sensitive, inflamed canal is desecrated on all hands, though part of a house not made with hands--a house that should be a home for the soul of man.

CHAPTER XVII.

COSTIVENESS.

The words constipation, obstipation and costiveness are often employed as if of exactly similar meaning, but it is well to let each stand for a particular condition. Obstipation implies that the canal of the intestine is stopped up or closed. Constipation carries the idea that the canal is completely filled up with refuse matter. In the normal condition the intestine is divided by transverse bulges or valves or dams into a number of separate segments, the entire arrangement having the effect of preventing too rapid descent of the feces. These folds within the canal may become too much narrowed by disease and thus prevent the movement of the matters inside; this is obstipation. Constipation, stuffing of the gut, may be the result of neglecting the call of nature, and after a time the ability to recognize and answer it is lost; or it may result from inflammation which itself comes from the bad habit mentioned.

The author prefers to use the term costiveness for the general debased condition of the system from auto-intoxication depending upon proctitis and similar conditions of the intestinal tract. And it must be remembered that the same patient may have two or more of these conditions at the same time. Constipation, obstipation and diarrhea may alternate through the progress of the case.

We would expect people suffering from constipation or obstipation to pass as fairly well people for a time, but the same is not true of patients having the other condition, costiveness. As we may speak of the stages of a disease like consumption, so we may speak of these three conditions as different stages of one affliction, the worst being costiveness with its progressive self-poisoning by the products of intestinal decomposition. Early in the case the system may pass these poisons out of the body with comparative ease, by way of the lungs, skin and kidneys. In time the second stage begins to make itself apparent, vitality becomes less and less, calling for a greater variety of medicines to correct the condition, as in the second stage of consumption, and also to arrest the progress of emaciation and anemia or anemic obesity.

The third stage of auto-intoxication is a most unhappy one. The impoverished tissues offer a most favorable soil for the development of diseased conditions. These three stages which are clear to the experienced eye of the physician may to the patient seem to be indistinguishable, the one from the other; and it must not be forgotten that the three conditions do not mean simply that a smaller or larger part of the intestine is clogged by its contents, but that the whole system is involved as well.

It cannot indeed be otherwise with the rapid circulation of the blood, nor need it excite wonder that such patients are thin and debilitated by the deadening of the powers of absorption, assimilation and elimination.

As a rule the many thin and puny infants and children of either sex, with bony points well exposed under a tightly drawn skin, which latter is clay-colored and pimply; children with headache and languor, without healthy interest in either studies or play;--these are the victims of intestinal poisoning as described. If they have inherited a spare habit of body from their parents such bodily ills will manifest themselves the more quickly. They ought to be fat and hearty as are the young of animals, but alas many are not! When the young animal is spare, a few days of rest with good diet will put flesh on it, demonstrating that the state of the bowels and the powers of assimilation are intact. Why does not man take on flesh in a similar way?

If the intelligent animals could talk, they would undoubtedly make all manner of fun of the intestinal canals which they see walking about, with a little flesh here and there seemingly by accident, and a skin which is clay-colored or jaundiced, anemic or flabby, the owner of it all poisoning himself by decomposition in his intestines!

CHAPTER XVIII.

INFLAMMATION.

If we desire to get a general idea of the changes that occur in an organ when it becomes inflamed, we must first have a knowledge of the normal structure of that organ, even though that knowledge be but superficial. Taking the intestines, for example, we see under the microscope that they are composed of layers of different tissues, called connective, epithelial, muscle, and nerve tissue; the first two forming a large part of the structure.

In the connective (and fatty) tissues a great many blood-vessels are found (varying in different parts of the organ), the existence of which is necessary for the production of inflammation, since at the very outset of the process, a discharge (or exudation) takes place from these blood-vessels, accompanied by changes or degenerations in the other kinds of tissue.

The process of inflammation is commonly associated with symptoms of heat, redness, swelling and pain, in greater or less degree, combined with which a change in the function of the organ is soon noticed. Micro-organisms are considered the primary cause of inflammation in many or even in most cases in which mechanical or chemical influences may undoubtedly be responsible primarily; and then again, each of these causes may be either external--that is, may originate from the outside world--or internal, that is, may be produced in and by the body itself.

The first pronounced change occurring in an organ under inflammation is an increase in the rapidity with which the blood circulates through the vessels--a so-called hyperemia--which soon gives place to a diminution (stasis) in the current together with an exudation from the blood-vessels; the latter is due to changes in the structure of their walls. This exudation soon occasions a cloudiness of the connective tissues and at the same time a desquamation (shedding in scales) of the epithelia (cells of the thin mucous surface). An irritation of the nerves also takes place.

The varieties of inflammation can be best apprehended by considering the different characters of the exudation. The exudation may be watery (called serous) or dense, the latter either fibrinous or albuminous. With a serous exudation there is swelling of the connective tissue and a desquamation of epithelia--the latter usually slight in character--which constitutes what is known as a catarrh; while with a fibrinous or albuminous exudation there is usually more or less destruction of the tissue itself, when, for example, we have "croup" or "diphtheria."

When the changes in the epithelia are only slight and secondary, it is spoken of as an interstitial (lying between) inflammation, which strictly speaking denotes confined to connective tissue, and is therefore a term not entirely correct. When the inflammation of the epithelia is severe and may lead to their partial destruction, it is called a parenchymatous inflammation; that is, one involving the soft cellular substance. There is still another variety, the suppurative, which is the most intense of all, and indicates the production of an abscess and the entire destruction of the tissue implicated.

Beside these general grades of inflammation there are special sorts produced by specific micro-organisms. In all general inflammation we may expect to find such organisms, which in most cases belong to the class of micrococci, such as staphylococci and streptococci. In gonorrhea we have a special organism called the "gonococcus"; while in tuberculosis--a variety of inflammation in which the blood-vessels are completely destroyed and a change or degeneration called "cheesy" is produced, leading to the production of a tubercle--a rod-like bacillus is invariably found, the well-known and unfortunately too common tubercle bacillus. In syphilis--another special variety of inflammation--a specific micro-organism is also surely present, but of this microbe science has not as yet discovered the exact nature.

The question of the origin of tumors or new growths is also an extremely important one; and it is undoubtedly true that many tumors arise where there was a previous inflammation, this being especially the case in tumors of the rectum. Why such a growth should arise in some cases and not in others is as yet unknown, though microbes are held by many to play an important role.

When an inflammation has lasted for such a length of time that it has become chronic, a new tissue will sooner or later be produced in varying amount; and this newly formed fibrous connective tissue may entirely replace previous normal structures. Through the exudation and consequent changes in the normal tissue a large amount of mucus is at first secreted, but this secretion becomes less and less marked the more the inflammation causes a desquamation of the epithelia. Pronounced desquamation with new formation of connective tissue and no fresh exudation will, sooner or later, occasion dryness--this dryness being sometimes very pronounced. The longer the inflammation lasts, the severer it will be; and the greater the amount of tissue it attacks, the more will the normal tissue be destroyed and replaced by a new connective tissue. A partial destruction will cause shrinkage of the organ (so-called "cirrhosis"); while a complete destruction of certain parts will result in what is known as "atrophy" (a wasting away of normal tissue). In atrophy the blood-vessels as well as the original connective and epithelial tissue are destroyed; while the newly formed tissue leads to hypertrophy (excessive over-growth) of other portions of the organ. Such a hypertrophy must not be confounded with an induration that may be present later, or even at the very commencement of an inflammation, due to modification of the blood-vessels and surrounding tissues.

Chronic inflammation, sooner or later, leads to secondary degenerations, that is, new products of the protoplasm, the most common of which is fatty degeneration. In this form fat granules and globules arise, which are at first minute, later on larger; these in certain organs, such as the liver, may become so pronounced as to entirely replace the original tissue. Another degeneration--which, however, is found only in chronic systemic disturbances, such as tuberculosis or syphilis--is the waxy or amyloid degeneration, a peculiar chemical change the exact nature of which is unknown.

Various chemical changes are by no means uncommon.

An important question is the decision as to the length of time an inflammation has lasted; and this at best can be determined only approximately and after long experience. The older the inflammation, the more the connective tissue has developed; this connective tissue is at first soft, but soon becomes more and more dense; the result being a varying degree of hardness of the organs.

Again, secondary degenerations are more pronounced in long-standing processes. In comparatively fresh cases blood-vessels are still more or less numerous and the tissue appears red, while in older cases these vessels become completely obliterated, and the tissues take on a white, glistening color, becoming harder and denser as the years advance. If a process has lasted twenty or thirty years, the changes to the eye and touch are practically the same as after forty or sixty years.

The changes, as here described, will be the same upon any mucous membrane; and in the large intestine can be easily studied and are perfectly characteristic.

Rarely does an infant escape repeated attacks of inflammation of the integument of the anus and the mucous membrane of the anal canal. The inflamed integument is treated and healed, but no attention is given to the inflamed mucous membrane so that the inflammation in time becomes chronic, involving the rectum also. Should the infant be so fortunate as to escape inflammation (proctitis) of these organs during the wearing of the diaper, there are numerous other exciting causes of inflammation which it will not be likely to escape, hence the almost universal symptom of constipation among civilized people; and hence later in life you hear the familiar expression, "I have a touch of the piles," and many other complaints of bowel ailments that are usually the outcome of that deplorable inflammation.

I have endeavored to make clear the fact that inflammation destroys normal tissues and blood-vessels, and that the newly formed tissue is cicatricial in character, that is poor in cells and vessels, with a tendency to contraction which of course lessens the bore of the gut. When the hypertrophy or thickening is extensive the appearance of the mucous membrane suggests the addition of one or more thicknesses of a chamois skin added to the inner surface of the anal and rectal canals. The hypertrophied or newly formed tissue may be limited to the rectum, leaving the anal tissues comparatively exempt from the superabundant cicatricial formation; or the hypertrophy may involve, to quite a degree, only the anal tissues and the integument around the anal orifice. The added connective tissue about the anus forms the skin into tabs, or into a circle of elongated integument around the orifice, with a mucous lining. These hypertrophied tabs or folds, like pruritus ani, are symptoms of proctitis.

Proctitis (the inflammation of the anal and rectal canals) is the most common and serious disease that afflicts man. The system is not only poisoned by bacteria and filth through proctitis, but proctitis is also the cause of the many annoying and painful local symptoms, such as hypertrophy, piles, abscess, fistula, cancer, polypus, fissure, pruritus, etc.

When the subject of proctitis is better understood by laymen they will see to it that the rectums of children receive an examination before the children are six years old, and thus obviate the necessity of dosing them with all sorts of medicine that follow improper diagnosis.

CHAPTER XIX.

PROCTITIS AND PILES.

Piles (hemorrhoids) are not the result of either the normal or abnormal growth of the tissues of the anal and rectal mucous membrane. They are developed by the combination of pathological and physiological conditions: (1) chronic inflammation or proctitis; (2) stricture of the anal canal and lower portion of the rectum, which may be spasmodic, or more or less permanent, which stricture pinches or constricts the canal, thereby inhibiting the circulation of the blood; (3) the pressure or straining effort during the act of defecation, occasioned by the constricted canal, which effort brings on greater local congestion and constriction of the tissues.

Pile formations are a symptom of chronic proctitis of fifteen, twenty or more years duration. Proctitis (inflammation of the anus or rectum) and periproctitis (inflammation of the connective tissue about the rectum) are by no means uncommon inflammatory processes. The mucous membrane like the skin is liable to injury or poisons and especially so at the orifices of the body. Let inflammation set in: if it be not cured at once, it will invade the canal, especially a canal like the rectum; in which case it will establish itself throughout from six to ten inches of its length, sometimes taking in the sigmoid flexure and even the colon. Just how long chronic inflammation confines itself to the mucous membrane before invading the areolar or lace-like connective tissue and the muscular tissue of the organ, I am unable to state.

The first symptom or indication that all the tissues are involved in the inflammatory process will most naturally be constipation. You have observed that inflammation of a portion of the skin on the arm, trunk or leg does not disturb the muscular movements of the region involved, except when the muscles underneath the skin are affected also, as in the case of deep burns where the movements are very much disturbed by the irritability, soreness and contraction of the diseased muscles. There is also an adhesive product excreted from the inflamed tissue that binds the muscular fibres of an organ together, and you have contraction of the organ and its usefulness impaired. Now, as this is precisely the pathological or diseased condition which chronic cases of proctitis and periproctitis present, you will readily understand how spasmodic and partial stricture or contraction occurs in the sore muscles (circular and longitudinal) of the anus and rectum. The length and the bore of the canal are diminished, and thus the circulation of the blood arrested by the pressure or gripping of the contracted muscles. This congestion of the blood brings about an anatomical change in the structure of the mucous membrane, which we call piles: a mere symptom of inflammation.

Medical authors have defined inflammation as follows: "(1) A series of changes constituting the local reaction to injury; (2) a series of changes that constitute the local attempt at repair of actual or referred injury of a part; (3) a series of local phenomena that are developed in consequence of primary lesion of the tissues and that tend to heal these lesions; (4) the method by which an organism attempts to render inert the noxious elements introduced from without or arising within it; (5) a disturbance of the mechanism of nutrition of an organ or tissue, affecting the structures concerned in its function."

These effects or changes give rise to the five cardinal symptoms of inflammation: pain, heat, redness, swelling and impaired function (dolor, calor, rubor, tumor, functio la).

Proctitis may exist many years before the pain and heat become noticeable or are complained of by the victim of this insidious disease, the bodily symptoms of which are well expressed before the local trouble demands attention and treatment. The sufferer from proctitis is unable to detect the change from a normal color of the mucous membrane (a light, muddy gray) to an extremely abnormal one (a fiery redness). The swelling or puffiness of the mucous membrane becomes more marked as repeated attacks of subacute and acute inflammation occur, from year to year, over a period of twenty or more years. During all this time impairment of the function and structure of the anal and rectal canals is incessantly going on. The nervous and muscular spasmodic contraction of the diseased anus and rectum, which in time become more or less permanently constricted, steadily increases the stagnation and engorgement of blood in the dilated arteries, veins, arterioles, venous rootlets and capillaries. All of the circulatory vessels, especially the smaller ones, become enlarged, varicose; and an aggregation of varicosed vessels forms a tumor called a pile or hemorrhoid. Inflammation interferes with nutrition of the anal and rectal tissues, rendering them friable or weak and easily broken; whence the bleeding and painful fissure or the anal ulcer, which so often are the outcome of proctitis and an accompaniment of piles.

As already stated, piles are one of the symptoms of proctitis, and all cases of piles involve more or less irritability and contraction of the anal canal and the terminal portion of the rectum through which the fecal matter is forced. All the muscular ability of the rectum, assisted by straining effort of the abdominal muscles, is concentrated upon the feces to force it through the constricted portion of the lower bowel. The force exerted not only develops pile tumors, but carries out with the feces those tumors that had reached considerable proportions; thus the frail diseased mucous membrane is torn, and another symptom added to a chronic disease. Observation for over twenty years has convinced me that chronic proctitis usually exists fifteen, twenty or more years before piles are developed (if developed at all), from daily pressure on the inflamed, congested, dilated, varicose, friable blood-vessels and surrounding tissue.

Piles are easily and quickly cured without any annoyance to the sufferer. Chronic proctitis may be cured, but not quickly, as time is required to undo damage to tissues so long invaded by inflammatory process. Any one that allows a continuance of "a touch of the piles," as the expression is, and omits to take proper treatment as soon as this "touch" is felt, simply invites or takes chances of some form of cancer of the lower bowel later in life.

All other forms of disease of the lower bowel will yield to treatment satisfactory to physician and patient, but I am sorry to say cancer cases are numerous, and up to the present time we have no cure for this dreadful disease. If you value health, if you desire to avoid future suffering and disease, be sure that the lower bowel is free from inflammation, for with such freedom you will escape the many symptoms of proctitis described in my treatise on diseases of the anus and rectum.

CHAPTER XX.

PRURITUS OR ITCHING OF THE ANUS.

One of the many symptoms of proctitis is the existence of anal channels from which an inflammatory product exudes through the skin, causing painful itching of the skin around the anal margin and not infrequently around the buttocks to the distance of three, six or even more inches from the anal orifice. An aggravated form of pruritus ani is much more trying to physical endurance than severe pain. Sometimes the torture is so great that a portion of the body will be covered with cold perspiration.

The natural color of the integument about the anus slowly changes to a dull whitish appearance. As the pathological process goes on, the skin becomes thickened and parchment-like. In exceptional cases the mucous membrane of the anal canal becomes toughened and hardened like cardboard. As a consequence there is a degree of inertia in the muscular action of the parts affected.

The inflamed, thickened and indurated integument near the anus takes on the form of folds, wrinkles or rug? of more or less prominence; but as these extend out over the buttocks they become more and more obliterated, leaving no clue to the direction of the channel which leads from the site of inflammation; which latter, however, may be learned from the itching, or from the burning sensation with some soreness, over portions of their length.

During a practice extending over twenty years, I have found only two cases in which one of these channels was the seat of a slight abscess. It is not usual that pus formations occur in these inflammatory channels. At the margin of the opening from the rectum to the anal tube are five or six small crescent-shaped loops, semi-lunar valves, separated by vertical ridges (the anal columns). Naturally in chronic proctitis the zone of tissue just above the sphincter muscles and slightly within their grasp at the upper portion of the anal tube, would suffer greatly from the morbid process, owing to the abnormal constriction of the tissues and to the incidental pressure and injury, from time to time, as the stool passes the diseased region. Just under the mucous membrane covering the anal columns and semilunar valves is the fatty tissue forming a bed upon which the mucous membrane rests. It is sufficiently lax to permit considerable movement of the mucous membrane on the muscular coat beneath it. The frail, fatty, loose connective tissue in the grasp of the sphincter muscles would be the first to become impaired by inflammatory process, the product of which finds its way down and out under the mucous membrane of the anal canal and integument of the buttocks for quite a distance, occasioning itching, pain, soreness or burning in the integument covering the course of the channel.

Here we have the pathological reason why local remedies to the outer surface of the skin will not cure pruritus ani. Also the reason why dieting is useless, and why internal remedies are worthless for the cure of anal itching; for the itching, as shown, is the result of an inflammatory product in the channels under the skin of the victim, numbering from five to twenty. Over fifteen years ago I discovered the cause of the great suffering from painful itching at the anus and contiguous tissues and have been able to give instant relief, and in a little time permanent cure, in every case treated since then. It is well for those who have an occasional attack of pruritus ani to take treatment at once for proctitis proper, as well as for this symptom, itching resulting from these channels. The proctitis, if neglected, will only be the means of increasing the size, length and number of these channels. In chronic, sub-acute and acute stages of proctitis there is more or less secretion of inflammatory product; and often the sufferer is able to discover, in dejections from the bowels, a yellow syrup-like fluid, of the consistency of glycerine or white of egg, at times streaked with blood and purulent matter indicating ulceration.

Should the proctitis be cured and these channels remain, there may be sufficient inflammatory product in the channels to ooze through the skin to the outer surface, and excite itching; or if a portion of the channel escapes treatment, the same symptom may be expected at any time.

The size and length of these channels are best determined by making a small opening into them through the integument, then inserting a silver probe in both directions, determining the distance under the mucous membrane of the anal tube and the distance under the skin of the buttocks.

In some cases a few of these channels open into the rectum just above the internal sphincter muscles and become filled with water during the use of the enema taken to move and cleanse the bowels. As a rule, one end of the channel is under the mucous membrane of the terminal portion of the rectum, and the other somewhere under the skin of the anus or of the buttocks.

I presume that no disease of the human body has been assigned more reasons for its existence, with the exception of constipation, than that mere symptom of a disease, anal pruritus; a symptom which "Regulars" call a "disease," but "Irregulars" know to be only a symptom. It is very amusing to observe how they fill pages in their text-books, guessing, wondering and paying their respects to the imaginary quack doctors, "who are reaping a harvest of ill-gotten gain." The usual medical writer is a compound of ignorance, egoism and garrulity, and this may account for the great crop of reasons for "diseases." However, the writers in question are not so much to blame after all, even though they do belong to county medical societies; for how can they well resist the literary itch with which most of them are afflicted? Let them keep on writing while victims of pruritus ani wear out their weary lives scratching through weary nights--nights that extend into years, until permanent invalidism seems to be their destiny and end. Who, verily, are the medical quacks? I will leave it to a jury composed of those who have been cured of pruritus ani.

I have yet to meet the first case of pruritus ani that is without the presence of the channels above described. There may be cases of itching at the anus and these channels entirely absent, but I have yet to discover such a case and

I very much doubt if it exists. I am happy to inform the reader that all cases of pruritus ani are cured with ease and without any restrictions as to diet, and without internal remedies for the blood, nervous system, etc., given by doctors that guess. The causes are easily discovered; the symptoms are easily found and removed; the victim of pruritus ani may therefore escape from the labyrinth of error of the medical authors and practitioners who ought to be educators instead of "obstacators"--obstacles and stumbling-blocks in medical progress.

CHAPTER XXI.

ABSCESS AND FISTULA.

In our daily affairs we take thought for the future and reason from cause to effect. We observe, anticipate, expect and suspect. This is a commendable practice, for it is the one that is most likely to lead to success. Can we not acquire a similar attitude and habit in regard to our health? Habit is subconscious attention. Can we not give sub-conscious attention to the little details of such bodily functions as are liable to get out of order? Can we not by a settled habit, that is, by the formation of a second nature, assure our vital success, on which the continuance of the enjoyment of life so much depends? If some part of a complicated machine gets out of order it must be repaired at once or damage may result to other parts of it. Again, if our business accounts will not balance, the error must be found and corrected at once, or the evidence of it will annoy us sooner or later. Why should not such prompt care and attention be given to the human mechanism, to the economy of vital functions? It is not often that we neglect disease of the hands, head, face or neck because the exposure of such disease to public gaze might embarrass us; but alas for the portion of the body out of sight, especially for the internal organs, when they fail to perform their functions normally. Most of us allow the mechanism of the human body to shift as best it can and as long as it can, should it happen to become ungeared, ignoring the frequent warnings which the ever increasing morbid changes and wreckage give us. And then we surrender and succumb. What else can we do?

Our vital creditors file their claims in the high court of Vital Bankruptcy. What poor business policy, and what a wretched tenant! For fifteen or more years we may have had warning "touches of the piles," sometimes accompanied with indigestion, constipation, diarrhea and insidious auto-infection and occasionally with local symptoms in and around the anal canal and its external orifice; these to an intelligent tenant should have been evidence of proctitis, or worse, of periproctitis--inflammation of the connective tissue of the rectal tube. What have we done? We have disregarded the warnings of our ungeared, disordered machine, or else we have merely tinkered with it. The human factory receives less attention than does the commercial. Soon, all too soon, the silver cord is loosed and the golden bowl broken, and just before that event, frightened, but too late, we do a little more tinkering under a doctor's direction, and spill the contents--of the golden bowl with which we were so careless--spill it into another world, to begin our folly over again!

Do you know that this occasional "touch of the piles" over a period of many years, and all that it involves, is a precursor and an invitation to the development of that deadly enemy, Cancer--a worse disaster than financial ruin? It is my duty to utter a warning here. Only one making a specialty of the diseases of the alimentary canal is aware of the frequency of the occurrence of cancer in the lower bowel resulting from chronic inflammatory process, induration, etc. I have been, again and again, shocked and alarmed at the reckless neglect that has brought on this as yet incurable disease--cancer.

These remarks apply well to what I have to say on Abscess and Fistula at the terminal portion of the intestinal canal. It is the old, old story of being "touched by the piles for many years," and neglect, ending in dread and despair at the necessity of being bored full of holes by pus seeking an outlet. The victim wonders at the spread of the local trouble, and that an opening for the pus canals has frequently to be made three to sixteen inches away from the seat of the abscess. In a former chapter the subject of proctitis and piles was gone into, and some idea given of the invasion of inflammation in the rectal and anal tissues.

In exceptional cases the exciting cause of anal and rectal abscess and fistula, or of abscess and fistula of the buttocks, may be a traumatic injury or accident, produced, say, by a blow or a fall bruising the tissues, or by sharp, hard substances--such as pieces of bone or nutshell--from within the canal, lacerating it. But wounds of this character are very infrequent compared with chronic inflammation (proctitis) as the exciting cause. There are several varieties of proctitis recognized as the exciting cause of abscess and fistula, namely, traumatic, dysenteric, diphtheritic, gonorrheal, catarrhal, etc. The reader should not only pardon me, but should be grateful if by adding another name to the list I point out the most common cause, namely, diaper-itic proctitis. As pointed out in the first chapter or two, the improper use of the diaper will evidence its deplorable result when the period of manhood or womanhood is reached, by some of the many symptoms of proctitis.

Proctitis may be considered as acute, subacute or chronic according to the duration of the process; or as atrophic or hypertrophic from the structural changes induced. But no matter about the cause and character of the proctitis, the question is, Have you inflamed anal and rectal canals? If you have, then the very annoying symptom, abscess or fistula, is liable to occur any day. Can you afford to take the chances?

Just under the mucous membrane of the anus and rectum there is a layer of loose, fatty, connective tissue, called areolar tissue. When it is invaded by inflammation, abscess and fistula may occur. On the outside of the rectal wall, at the terminal portion, there is also much loose, fatty (areolar) tissue filling the ischio-rectal fossa, which is very prone to suppuration, and inflammation here is called periproctitis. This is the most common and serious seat and source of the septic process, which process is usually the proximate cause of death after capital surgical operations upon the rectum. Beside the abundance of fatty tissue--whose function is to serve as a cushion to the rectum at its terminal portion and at the back and sides of the wall--there is a triangular space in front of the rectum containing fatty areolar tissue, which space is often the location of a pus cavity. Pus, like all fluids, follows the path of least resistance. The progress of imprisoned pus may take weeks, months and years before an abnormal communication between the abscess and the external portion of the body is completed. The imprisoned contents of the abscess cavity and the pus canal or fistula often give rise to much annoyance before finding an outlet. There will be pain in the muscles of the buttocks, called myalgia; and pain at the end of the spine, called coccygodynia. For this latter pain do not, I pray you, as is so often done, have your spine removed by the too ready surgeon. No need of it at all. You might just as sensibly have the muscles cut out for myalgia. Pus in fistulous channels may burrow for several years through the muscular and connective tissue structures before finally forming an external opening through the integument; although its nearness to the surface is frequently marked by a localized puffiness and inflammation, which, however, may disappear for a time without forming an external opening. This condition of affairs results in periodical attacks of coccygodynia, myalgia and neuralgia of the buttocks and lower extremities.

The important question with the victim of abscess and fistula is, "How did I get it? I don't care for the various and numerous names you give to these fistulas: what I should like to know is, How does it come about that I, an apparently healthy person, have such a nasty disease?" Simply years of neglect, is my answer. Neglect is due sometimes, and perhaps generally, to ignorance of the thing neglected. The laity can in large measure blame the medical profession for it, and especially those surgeons who have long made a specialty of the treatment of anal and rectal diseases.

CHAPTER XXII.

THE ORIGIN AND USE OF THE ENEMA.

Pliny recorded the fact that "the use of clysters or enemata was first taught by the stork, which may be observed to inject water into its bowels by means of its long beak." The British Medical Journal, reviewing the newly published Storia della Farmacia, says that Frederigo Kernot describes in it the invention of the enema apparatus, which he looks upon as an epoch in pharmacy as important as the discovery of America in the history of human civilization. The glory of the invention of this instrument, so beneficial to suffering mankind, belongs to an Italian, Gatenaria, whose name ought to find a modest place together with Columbus, Galileo, Gioja and other eminent and illustrious Italians. He was a compatriot of Columbus and professor at Pavia, where he died in 1496, after having spent several years in perfecting his instrument. The enema apparatus may be justly named the queen of the world, as it has reigned without a rival for three hundred years over the whole continent, besides Brazil and America. The enema came into use soon after the invention of the apparatus itself. Bouvard, physician to Louis XIII, applied two hundred and twenty enemata to this monarch in the course of six months. In the first years of Louis XIV it became the fashion of the day. Ladies took three or four a day to keep a fresh complexion, and the dandies used as many for a white skin. Enemata were perfumed with orange, angelica, bergamot and roses, and Mr. Kernot exclaims enthusiastically, "O se tornasse questa moda!" (Oh, that this fashion would return!). The medical profession at first hailed the invention with delight, but soon found the application infra dig., and handed it over to the pharmacist; but shameful invectives, sarcasms and epigrams, hurled at those who exercised the humble duty of applying the apparatus, made them at last resign it to barbers and hospital attendants. (Year Book of Therapeutics, Wood, 1872.)

"The history of the warm bath," says Dr. Paris, "presents another curious instance of the vicissitudes to which the reputation of our valuable resources is so universally exposed. That which for so many ages was esteemed the greatest luxury in health, and the most efficacious remedy in disease, fell into total disrepute in the reign of Augustus, for no other reason than because Antonius Musa had cured the Emperor of a dangerous malady by the use of the cold bath. The most frigid water that could be procured was in consequence recommended on every occasion.... This practice, however, was doomed but to an ephemeral popularity, for, although it restored the Emperor to health, it shortly afterward killed his nephew and son-in-law Marcellus, an event which at once deprived the remedy of its credit and the physician of his popularity.

"That the warm and not the cold bath was esteemed by the ancient Greeks for its invigorating properties may be inferred from a dialogue of Aristophanes, in which one of the characters says, 'I think none of the sons of the gods ever exceeded Hercules in bodily and mental force.' Upon which the other asks, 'Where didst thou ever see a cold bath dedicated to Hercules?'

"Thus there exists a fashion in medicine, as in the other affairs of life, regulated by the caprice and supported by the authority of a few leading practitioners, which has been frequently the occasion of dismissing from practice valuable medicines and of substituting others less certain in their effects and more questionable in their nature. As years and fashion revolve, so have these neglected remedies, each in its turn, risen again into favor and notice, whilst old receipts, like old almanacs, are abandoned until the period may arrive that will once more adjust them to the spirit and fashion of the times." (J. A. Paris, Pharmacologia, p. 31, New York, 1825.)

"A story told of Voltaire," says Dr. Arthur Leared, "well illustrates both the evil effects of constipation and the advantage of using the enema. The great philosopher was one day so miserable and dejected that he told a friend he had resolved to hang himself. His friend called the next morning to ascertain whether the resolve had been or was intended to be carried out. But Voltaire only replied, with a smile, 'I have been well washed out this morning.'" (Op. cit., p. 200.)

For those suffering from chronic intestinal uncleanliness or constipation, an occasional intestinal wash-out, or bath, is quite as satisfactory as an "occasional" external bath or the "occasional" use of a cathartic medicine. If there is a necessity for cleansing and purifying the bowels at all, why not do it properly and systematically until the condition that made the artificial cleansing necessary is removed? Who would tolerate the cleaning of dining-room, kitchen, dairy and other utensils in domestic use only when they became so foul that they could not be endured any longer without great annoyance? Away with the "occasional" cleansing habit for either external or internal bodily cleanliness! There are persistent causes for internal uncleanliness, for the tardy action of the bowels, which require regular periods for cleansing until cure is effected.

It is estimated that food taken into the stomach will reach the colon in five hours. For nineteen hours the sewage waste of the body is gradually becoming a fetid pool before an outlet is furnished it by the one-movement-a-day people; and O ye gods of health! how many of us there are that haven't even one movement a day! For a few hours the absorbent cells of the colon will try to extract as much of the nutritious residue as the system calls for, but along with it a lot of poisonous filth will be absorbed. The call of the system for nourishment should be fully answered by the small intestines. Savages have four or five movements a day, and we certainly should not have less than three. People of refined sentiments will, at such a disclosure, bestir themselves to better things.

Water, when properly applied, is the only remedy that meets the physiological and pathological requirements of the chronically constipated. By its use the diseased, spasmodically contracted muscular tube is simply dilated, and the imprisoned feces and gases above are permitted to pass down and through the temporarily occluded section of the diseased bowels, the patient will have the consciousness of neatly accomplishing an imperative requirement, and the satisfaction which cleanliness entails.

CHAPTER XXIII.

HOW OFTEN SHOULD AN ENEMA BE TAKEN?

The following lines will show you how advertising is done in medical journals. "Dear Doctor: The spring being the time for cathartics, I beg to call your attention to R. L. (yellow label),..."

Why is spring a special time for cathartics? Has the intestinal canal been obstructed like the Erie Canal during the winter months? With as much propriety they might advertise: "Dear Doctor: The spring being the time for bathing, I beg to call your attention to antiseptic bath soap,..."

I suppose that a sort of annual cleansing of the alimentary canal is suggested so that the summer heat may be less objectionable, as it warms up foul bodies. However, attention once a year is better than none at all, as said of the Augean stables.

Not long ago I had a conversation with the proprietor of a bath cabinet company, who had given some thought to hygienic measures, and he considered it essential to flush the bowels with water once a month to secure "proper cleanliness." This opinion is quite in advance of the annual cathartic cleansing. Some people may have acquired the habit of a monthly cathartic "cleansing"; others wash out once a week, and a few once a day: all of them act from their idea of cleanliness, as they would perform the ablution of their hands, face and body. There are some hygienic students who have adopted the idea of "cleansing" the bowels with warm water once or twice a week, which practice is quite in advance of the annual or monthly attention. All have reasons for the manner and time they adopt to "cleanse" the bowels; and yet they find that they are not cleansed properly, as they still have spells of biliousness and misery. They wonder at themselves for being so rash and bold as to take an enema twice a week, and begin to feel that they have reached a point of positive danger.

One anxiety is that they will weaken the bowels by the use of a pint or a quart of water once a month, or once or twice a week. Another is that they will wash away the mucus, leaving the membrane of the bowels as dry as an oven. Another is that they will form the dreadful habit of using the enemata. What a pity to form such a cleanly habit! Sorry for them!

Another stubborn objection is, that flushing of the bowels is not natural. These foolish objections and fears can be attributed to medical authors who belong to medical societies. It is very strange how these authors adopt so many wrong notions about the physiology and pathology of the bowels. What an erroneous and absurd idea that the enema should weaken the bowels! Why should it? Exercise ought to strengthen muscular tissue; and what could give the bowels more gentle muscular exercise than the proper use of them? Has the reader any idea of the amount of water requisite for the distention of an elastic muscular tube, about five feet in length and two and a half inches in diameter in the widest part? The large intestine is capable of great distention, as is frequently demonstrated in fecal impaction described in previous chapters. The quantity is named in gallons. The amount of water usually injected at one time--from one pint to two quarts--can hardly be said to distend the bowels at all. I wish the enemata did have power to weaken that part of the bowel involved in disease. I am very sorry it does not weaken it. For twenty years it has been demonstrated to my mind that almost every case of chronic constipation, biliousness, intestinal foulness, diarrhea, indigestion, self-poisoning (auto-infection or auto-intoxication) was due to too much activity and vigor of the lower bowels, this excessive activity and vigor being the result of chronic proctitis, colitis, etc. To lessen this muscular irritability, and to devise means to relieve and cure quickly, has cost me more studious hours than the aggregate of all the other diseases and symptoms of the lower bowels.

If liquids washed away the mucus from the mucous membrane, the throats of many individuals ought to be very harsh and dry, inasmuch as six to eight glasses of liquids pass through their mouths and throats during every day of twenty-four hours. Even after the "dry feeling in the throat and stomach" has been bountifully attended to by the owner, the conversation usually becomes more loquacious and hilarious, and there is no suggestion that the intemperate person had spent many hours in a hot desert without water. The frequent flushings they give their throats and stomachs really do not seem to wash the mucus away.

When a person consults an oculist about an affection of the eyes and glasses are prescribed, good sense will inform him that the glasses must be worn while the imperfect functioning of the eyes requires them. If a limb be fractured and splints be applied, would you worry lest you form the habit of wearing them? Certainly not; you expect in due time to recover the proper use of the limb. So if you are compelled to use crutches you do not worry about forming the crutch habit, for you will use them as long as needed and discard them at the proper time.

As to its being unnatural to flush the bowels with water, I would say that it is very unnatural to suffer from proctitis accompanied with its annoying symptoms, such as constipation, indigestion, diarrhea, auto-intoxication, emaciation, anemia, muddy complexion, foul breath, blotches and pimples on the face, each and all of which indicate a physical debasement.

It is unnatural to wear glasses, crutches, splints, wigs, artificial teeth, artificial eyes, but many people do such unnatural things. Many of our habits are not exactly "natural," but they are rational, none the less; such, for example, as bathing the body night and morning; cleansing the mouth and teeth after each meal; and the nostrils and ears several times a day. The frequency of these practices may, with some people, be unnecessary and useless, but no real harm is done by their scrupulous cleanliness--physical and mental.

Proctitis is usually worse than it seems to be. This is because of the insidious progress of the inflammation during the fifteen, twenty or more years before the local symptoms at the anus or in the anal canal are sufficiently annoying to compel the sufferer to seek treatment. Such sufferers are, as a rule, born with the idea that the liver regulates the whole alimentary canal; and if the sufferer has not this hereditary notion, his physician will soon impart it to him with his diagnosis and treatment. The disciple of cathartics, whether the cathartics be in the form of pills, powders, or solutions, or contain belladonna and opium to overcome the cramping pain the dose would otherwise occasion, has no legitimate reason to indulge in the hope of a cure or of even moderate relief of the real source of trouble--the proctitis. It is proceeding on the liver theory, when the key is, as has been shown in these articles, Proctitis, inflammation of the anus and rectum. Physicians ignorant of the key to all bowel troubles even prescribe strychnine in order to stimulate bowels which have already an excessive amount of stimulation due to the presence of the proctitis, which, as has been said, over-stimulates the lower bowels because of the inflammation.

The chronic character of proctitis of many years' duration, improperly diagnosed and treated, must necessarily compel a rather long and continued use of the enema, especially so if not accompanied by proper local treatment of all the inflamed surface. I should not care to treat patients suffering from proctitis, constipation, etc., unless they used the enema twice a day. The feces and gases should escape the bowels at least twice in twenty-four hours. Any less than two stools a days is abnormal and will result in infection and disease. You may not always succeed in having two stools when first treating the local disease, but what you properly start out to accomplish will be attained in due time.

Free evacuation of the contents of the bowels should occur at least twice in twenty-four hours. This can be accomplished by injecting into the colon from one to four quarts of warm water. Before taking the large injection, relieve the bowels of any gas seeking liberation, and of course, also, of whatever feces may come readily. Then take a small injection, using very little water: just enough to bring on a relief of as much feces and gas as possible. It is not well to drive the gas back and up into the colon; hence the precaution to suggest a further passage with a small quantity of water before taking the large injection.

Enemata, and also the use of the recurrent douche, can in no way be harmful--if the water be of a proper temperature--to a normal or even to a diseased bowel; therefore the fear of habit is absurd and should not receive a moment's consideration. The length of time during which the enemata and the douche are to be used, whether months or years, will depend on the character of the disease that made its use necessary.

CHAPTER XXIV.

MAN'S BEST FRIEND.

Travel the world from end to end You ne'er will find a better friend Than sparkling water, pure and free, Most precious boon to you and me. It cheers the faint, it crowns the feast, Makes food to grow for man and beast; In sickness soothes the fevered frame, There's healing in its very name. And what can more life-giving be Than cooling breezes from the sea, Whose bosom bears upon their way The stately ships from day to day? A treasure trove of priceless worth; A jewelled belt for mother Earth, Encircling with its silvery bands, She binds together many lands. To cure disease dame Nature brings Her remedy in mineral springs; Water without, water within, Equally good for stout or thin; And more than man can e'er devise Invigorates and purifies. Travel the world from end to end, You ne'er will find a better friend.

CHAPTER XXV.

PHYSIOLOGICAL IRRIGATION.

The scientific irrigation of land is pretty well understood by those who have financial interest in soil requiring it. The wonderful beauty and freshness of flower and fruit give evidence of what scientific irrigation can do. So from a commercial and esthetic point of view the proper amount of daily moisture for land, tree or vine, is of such importance that it receives the consideration of those interested. How many persons, however, in the course of a lifetime have given ten minutes to serious consideration of the question: How much water should be imbibed daily under the varying conditions of the body's garden? Those who give no consideration to the problem of how to attain and maintain a healthy and vigorous physical basis are persons who usually drift into habits for which they will, sooner or later, have to pay the penalty.

For the first twenty or more years the body is, as a rule, unfortunate in not having an intelligent tenant. For man misuses his physiological estate, and lets things go to rack and ruin ere he wakes to realize how it might have been as to length of days and strength of body and mind. Enlighten him, after he has reached adult years, on the values and needs of physiological and psychological functions; you will find that however eager he may be to follow the light he is handicapped by vicious habits and by confirmed, destructive changes which had seized on him when he was quite too young and incompetent to care for his body. What a topsy-turvy world this is, to be sure!

It is astonishing what a number of people there are who drink little or nothing, and especially amazing is it to find this lack of sense in people suffering from constipation. One would suppose that they above all others would see the wisdom of irrigating their bowels. But it is seldom that there is one who thinks of such a thing. A cup of coffee or tea at meal-time, in addition to the liquid contained in the food, is the extent of water consumption by ever so many teetotalers and other "totalers," especially women, until they reach, say, thirty years of age. Such persons as a rule are not long-lived, inasmuch as their power of resistance is small, owing to their lack of blood, a lack in quality as well as in quantity. The blood pressure in their arteries and veins is light, as evidenced by their pale, sallow complexion, and the dry, scaly, feverish skin, which seldom or never perspires. The body garden has not been properly irrigated and is slowly drying up as age advances. Did you ever notice how like death such persons appear when they are asleep? Their dull, pasty complexions alarm us then. When I see them a desire to soak these dried specimens of humanity possesses me. Is it not unfortunate that we were not born with an automatic irrigator? We even lack a tube on our boiler to indicate the danger point! Deficient by nature in these little conveniences, and unaided by science, man is compelled to give some attention to the irrigation of his physiological soil, however indifferent or careless he may be.

Planters and gardeners have treatises on irrigation. Have mothers or nurses any similar guides? Such books are unknown to modern civilization. Infants, boys and girls, and adults are brought up haphazard, and their garden of life becomes choked with weeds. The drought soon makes itself felt, and a little graveyard mound is their usual fate. Before some of us wither and fade, to what a pest-weed is our adipose changed for want of life-giving water.

Man's most serious physiological fault is the toleration of constipation; or even of semi-constipation induced by the twenty-four-hour habit of stooling. In other words, his fault is the toleration of intestinal uncleanliness. And next to this foolhardiness is his negligence in the matter of drinking daily a quantity of pure soft water sufficient to aid in the proper stimulation and circulation of the blood, in the proper elimination of the waste material from the body, and in the proper assimilation of nutriment by the system.

If parents would encourage their children to become bibbers of pure spring water daily it would not be easy to make them bibbers of intoxicants in after years. I would give a child all the liquid it desires, I would even encourage it to take more rather than less, and the best liquid of all for this purpose is pure soft water. Man's body is 70 per cent water. It is therefore a good-sized water cask with a ramification of countless canals or pipes imbedded in soft connective tissues, nerves and muscles, all of which are supported by a bony framework; through the centre of this runs the alimentary canal, down which waters may flow and disappear like unto a stream lost in the sand, to reappear and ooze from skin, lungs, kidneys and intestinal canal. Every organ and tissue luxuriates in water; they lave and live in and by it. With all kinds of food it is introduced into the body. Water acts as a solvent for the nutritious elements and as a sponsor for the elimination of foreign substances and worn-out tissues of the system. It also serves to maintain a proper degree of tension in the tissues, which tension is essential to the proper circulation of the lymphatic fluids.

The tonic reaction of externally applied water is well known. But the advantages of the internal use of water are hardly known at all because the reactions of the circulation, temperature, respiration, digestion and secretions are less noticed.

Two or three pints of cold water at a temperature of forty to forty-five degrees drunk at intervals of half an hour will reduce the pulse from eight to thirty beats. The copious drinking of cold water will act as a diuretic, removing stagnated secretions, and will at the same time improve the quality of the pulse and the arterial tone. The drinking of warm water will increase the pulse from five to fifteen beats, and at the same time will relax the vessel walls and also increase the cutaneous secretions to a marked degree.

The drinking of a large quantity of water not only increases the secretions of the kidneys--assisting them in the work of carrying off solid constituents, especially urea--it also increases the secretions of the skin, saliva, bile, etc. Under proper conditions the internal use of water acts as a stimulant to the nerves that control the blood-vessels, a stimulant similar to that produced by its external application.

I advise the drinking of a copious quantity of water daily. There need be no fear that this practice will thin the blood too much, as the ready elimination of the water will not permit such a result to ensue. I would further advise the generous use of water (temperature 60? at meal-times. I pray you do not drink to wash down food: a bad habit of most of us. Drink all you desire; and if you are like many who have no desire for water, cultivate it, even if it takes years. The imbibed water will be in the tissues in about an hour; and the entire quantity will escape in about three and one-half hours. The demand on the part of the system for water is subject to great variation and is somewhat regulated by the quantity discharged from the organism. Physiologists declare that water is formed in the body by a direct union of oxygen and hydrogen, but those who have cultivated the drink-little habit need not hope to find an excuse for themselves in this fact: chronic ill-health betrays them. Water in organic relations with the body never exists uncombined with inorganic salts (especially sodium chloride) in any of the fluids, semi-solids, or solids of the body. It enters into the constitution of the tissues, not as pure water, but always in connection with inorganic salts. In case of great loss of blood by hemorrhage, a saline solution of six parts of sodium chloride with one thousand parts of sterilized water injected into the system will wash free the stranded corpuscles and give the heart something to contract upon.

When water is taken into the stomach, its temperature, its bulk, and its slight absorption react upon the system; but the major part of it is thrown into the intestinal canal. When it is of the temperature of about 60?it gives no very decided sensation either of heat or cold; between 60?and 45?it creates a cool sensation, and below 45?a decidedly cold one. Water at a temperature of about 50?is a generator of appetite. A sufficient quantity should be taken for that end; say, one or two tumblers an hour or so before each meal, followed by some exercise. Those who have acquired the waterless habit, and the many ills resulting from it, will hardly relish cool water as an appetizer; but if they would become robust they must adopt the water habit--a habit that will refresh and rejuvenate nature.

Water of a temperature between 60?and 100?relaxes the muscles of the stomach and is apt to produce nausea, especially if the effect of bulk be added to that of temperature. Lukewarm water seems to excite an upward peristalsis of the intestines and thus produces sickness.

Hot water acts as a stimulant and antiseptic, as a sedative and as a food. Water at a temperature of 110?to 120? or more, will nearly always relieve a foul stomach and intestines. It should be slowly sipped, so that the stomach may not be uncomfortably distended. After imbibing a pint or a pint and a half, wait for fifteen or thirty minutes to give it time to pass into the bowels, then drink more if thought advisable. Drink it an hour before meal-time. It will excite downward peristalsis, will dilute the foul contents of the stomach, and will thus aid the escape of these contents into the intestines, which latter require the washing process as well. Sometimes it is a good thing to omit one, two or three meals while the washing process is being continued. Commence treatment with pure hot water. To make it appetizing, add a pinch of salt or of bicarbonate of soda; with children add sugar. It will pay you to follow this treatment for the cleansing of the alimentary canal.

The vitality of the body may be sustained for days and weeks on water alone; there is therefore no hurry about food. If human beings would only keep their bowels and stomachs clean they would avoid all the ills that flesh is heir to, except, of course, those due to accident.

My remarks have been confined to irrigation per orem (that is, by way of the mouth), and nothing has been said of irrigation per anum (by injection), since I have treated the latter subject fully in several previous chapters, to which the reader is referred. Be sure to follow the counsel there given, and use the enema two or three times a day in moderate quantities as indicated.

CHAPTER XXVI.

PROPER TREATMENT FOR DISEASES OF THE ANUS AND RECTUM VERY ESSENTIAL.

No doubt the readers of the preceding chapters on proctitis and its numerous symptoms--noted under separate headings--would like to know something about the home treatment for such an insidious and grave disease. Every sufferer wants to be a self-doctor. This commendable desire it is usually impossible to put into practice. If physicians so often fail to cure the ailments I have described, what can be expected of those who have no knowledge at all of diagnosis and treatment?

A skilful physician is the choicest gem of civilization, and an intelligent patient its worthy setting. Surely it is a moral crime, an inexcusable folly to tolerate a disease with its inevitable train of dire consequences, up to the point when the discomfort compels one to seek treatment. There are patients, of course, who have good and sufficient excuses for their painful predicament; they have, for example, tried persistently for relief and cure, but have failed to find a physician competent to treat their particular case. How many unskilled prescribers there are, and how glaring their shortcomings! Some hold out taking inducements to sufferers; their one object being to transfer their patients' cash to their own pocket. 'Twere charitable to consider these ignorant; but alas! many of them are poisoned by the "fakir" germ. Stuff is sold by the conscienceless, claiming to cure "piles," to "give instant relief," and promising "a complete cure in a few days"; and as to itching piles, why! "only a few applications are necessary for a cure; six boxes for five dollars"! etc.

No remedy that sufferers apply themselves can be more than a temporary relief: it cannot really cure piles, polypus, fistula, tabs, pruritus (itching)--all of them consequences of proctitis. Of course one should be thankful for the little relief to be got temporarily from advertised and drug-store drugs; nothing more than relief can be expected of them. There are indeed times when a palliative treatment will serve to tide the sufferer over a few days until he is able to consult a competent physician. But how strange it is that so many sufferers regard their anatomy and physiology so lightly as to think of using remedies, even for relief, without first undergoing a thorough examination by a competent physician. In troubles of a rectal character it is exceedingly foolhardy to allow any one to prescribe without insisting upon a thorough examination to ascertain whether there be any disease of a cancerous nature present, or what the trouble actually is, and its progress. To expect one remedy or prescription to meet all the requirements for the cure of a chronic disease of the anus and rectum and of the many complications accompanying it is hardly sensible, but that is just what a great many do expect. No one remedy in the market, or any number of them combined can effect a cure, for the simple reason that proper local treatment by a physician is of paramount importance. Unless of a traumatic (externally produced wound) origin, diseases of the anal and rectal canals are usually of fifteen, twenty or more years' incubation before the annoying symptoms become apparent. This accounts for the slight attention to the maturing trouble and for the fact that such attention can afford nothing more than a palliation or postponement. A real cure requires a combination of means, all working harmoniously for the proper length of time. Proper treatment and the proper time are the two prime requisites; and the third and final requisite is, of course, a sensible patient.

Before home treatment is to be thought of it is accordingly advisable to have an examination and a prescription for the specific local treatment necessary for a trouble like piles, fissure, polypus, tabs, itching, fistula, varicose veins, abscess, ulcer, granulation, hypertrophy, or atrophy as the case may be. The local treatment can best be aided by a combination of remedies with suitable instruments for their use between the periods of local attention by the physician. The writer of this has no cure-all to send the sufferers, although it might be to his financial advantage to have one; he is, however, always ready to advise and relieve those who cannot visit him immediately. The relief afforded often facilitates the cure by permitting a more extensive local treatment at the first visit.

The Use of Instruments for Injecting Water.

To do something at home for one's self for relief from soreness and pain due to anal and rectal diseases, a few suitable instruments are required with which specific remedies may be used, especially that excellent remedy--water.

It is unfortunate that the anal and rectal canals cannot be given rest when invaded by disease. Daily elimination of feces is a very important factor to health and to treatment. To accomplish this the very best means is water in various quantities as the case demands. It does not irritate the diseased canals--as cathartics do--but aids in the escape of imprisoned feces and gases which lodge above the region of the morbid process. Evacuation should be accomplished twice a day, by the injection at first of three or four quarts of water--thus obtaining a good daily flushing of one's sewer--and then, if advisable, gradually lessening the quantity at subsequent injections to one or two pints at a time. The temperature should be 100?to 105?or more. Some people have an idea that water at the temperature named has a remedial effect on an inflamed anus and rectum. It has none whatever; all it does is to wash away the deposits which might irritate the inflamed surface. Water at a temperature of 100?to 105?is not an especially good antiseptic; and its intestinal use should not be continued longer than to bring away the effete and fetid material which may be lodged in the colon, sigmoid flexure and rectum. In the majority of cases its use should be limited to aiding the feces to escape from their normal receptacle--the sigmoid flexure--whenever proctitis does not extend beyond the rectum. But many persons are deceived by the conduct of proctitis and are thus likely to omit the regular irrigation twice a day. They believe themselves to be in pretty good condition and do not realize that their old, implacable enemy may be excited into riot any day; in which case the insurrection may last for months and then slowly settle down to semi-quiet again, reaching finally the point of its best behavior for a short period or until again provoked.

The Use of the Recurrent Douche.

Water at a temperature of 120?to 130?properly applied is a good therapeutic agent in the treatment of proctitis. At that temperature it is an excellent antiseptic and astringent. Its continuous use for half to one hour applied with a recurrent douche brings about a contraction of the engorged and dilated blood-vessels; and accompanied by local treatment and by other remedies is the best means known for restoring the nerves to their normal function of controlling the proper circulation of blood in the diseased organ. Treatment with the recurrent douche is of course to follow, not to precede, the evacuation of the bowels; but at any time when there is a tendency toward additional evacuation on the admission of the hot water, the new douche is easily adjustable to the contingency without removal from the anal canal; it will facilitate the escape of the feces with the return flow of the water. The new recurrent douche has therefore the great advantage of promoting simultaneously both the thorough evacuation of the bowels, and the therapeutic effect of hot water.

Sitz-Bath.

There are patients who, because of years of neglect of their local ailments, are taken with severe attacks of inflammation of the anus and rectum, involving considerable prolapse, much swelling around the anus, and general local soreness and pain; all of which is often accompanied by a general disrelish of life. For this condition nothing is so good as a very hot sitz-bath, if properly adjusted to the parts and continued for about an hour at a sitting. The alleviation afforded is so decided and the local and prolonged application of hot water so restorative that it may be left to the sufferer to determine how often this bath is to be repeated. It may be taken as often as there is an inclination to do so. The sitz-bath apparatus should be scientifically adapted to the parts so that the bather will not sit lower than ten or twelve inches, thereby avoiding a straining position. During the bath there should be more or less pressure against the anal tissues, which assists the hot water in expelling the blood from the inflamed parts. From the beginning to the end of the bath the water must be as hot as the tissues will tolerate. Only a small portion of the buttocks need be immersed in the hot water.

Spring Water the Ideal Beverage.

Those who suffer from disease of the rectum, with rare exceptions, are constipated or semi-constipated, which condition in turn aggravates or disturbs the inflamed parts. To overcome this constipated condition all sorts of laxatives are taken, which will in the end do grave harm not only to the whole system, but especially to the inflamed parts, irritating them still more. There is a valuable therapeutic agent seldom taken by the constipated; in fact, it is never thought of; unfortunately the remedy is not easily to be had in its pure state by most of us, boxed as we are in cities. Sold under various names as mineral water, it is too often adulterated. 'Tis a simple remedy, and yet it has a wider range of healing power than any other; a universal solvent, applicable to all diseases and all states of health. I would write it at the head of all remedial agents: pure spring water! We do not drink enough water. If we were to imbibe at least two quarts of pure water daily we would be healthier and have better movements of our bowels. Water may be taken freely during mealtime; not, however, for the purpose of washing down half-masticated food. Alcoholic drinks, coffee and tea would better be dispensed with, also tobacco. The nervous system has enough to bear without the use of avoidable irritants.

Other Hygienic Agencies.

Too much cannot be urged as to the advisability of a proper amount of exercise, sleep, rest, food, breathing, cleanliness (internal and external), as well as and above all, pure, high-minded thoughts and serene temper--the outcome of the habit of viewing life philosophically. Care should be taken to protect the feet and body from sudden climatic changes, thus avoiding catarrhal troubles, especially of the lower bowels.

As to the wise and proper use of nature's pharmacopoeia, nothing need be said here. However, I may be within my limits when I advise patients to use a little sense and not neglect disease of the lower bowel any more than they would neglect that of the eye, ear and throat. In the latter case they submit at once to an examination. Why not in the former? Let them bear in mind that the cure of chronic proctitis is no holiday job; that it is, on the contrary, a task which requires constant attention. To merely relieve the annoying symptoms that accompany it cannot be called a cure. But on the other hand relief may be the commencement of a cure. Of course the true way of looking at the subject of this disease is to regard the cure of proctitis as necessarily leading to the disappearance in time of all the other troubles that were the outcome of that ailment. Through the harmonious efforts of patient and physician, marvellous results are often obtainable.

CHAPTER XXVII.

THE BODY'S BOOK-KEEPING.

Man's food is as varied as his work, more varied than the climate, with one food for the luxurious and one for the poor. The majority of us take what we can get, making no complaints; even when we have a cook and a good one the same is true. The ideal diet prepared by the ideal cook no one has as yet made fashionable, but one thing is within the reach of all--cleanliness of the sewers of the body. Keep the contents of the bowels moving down and out steadily and regularly and you may eat almost any food and in almost any preparation and still be healthy.

Just as a steam-engine, running at a given rate of speed, must be supplied with fuel sufficient to maintain that speed, so the human body must have the requisite food to maintain the speed of civilized society and business, and replace the waste of the tissues; otherwise decline sets in and the reserve store of strength is exhausted. How shall we determine the proper amount and kind of food for the various ages, sexes, and conditions of life?

A leading authority says that the character and amount of the daily excreta furnish suggestions as to the required food supply. (Kirk's Physiology, p. 208.) These excreta are found to be carbon, nitrogen, hydrogen, oxygen in great part, with some sulphur, phosphorus, chlorine, sodium, etc. A summary is given (ibid., p. 432) of the expenditure for twenty-four hours:

1. From the lungs: Carbonic acid about 15,000 grains Water " 5,000 "

2. From the skin: Water " 11,500 " Solid and gaseous matters " 250 "

3. From the kidneys: Water " 23,000 " Organic matter " 680 " Saline bodies " 420 "

4. From the intestines: Water " 2,000 " Organic and mineral substances " 800 "

Total daily expenditure: Solid matters " 17,150 " Water " 49,500 "

Altogether about eight and a half pounds.

The credit side of the sheet is about as follows:

Solids (chemically dry foods) " 8,000 grains Water, combined or otherwise 35,000 to 40,000 " Oxygen, absorbed by the lungs " 13,000 "

Altogether about eight and a half pounds.

With the proper balance between the intake and the outgo, the functions of the body will be carried on normally, but the balance must be a proper one;

that is, not only must the entire waste be repaired but the correct proportions of one kind of food and another must be observed. If all the elements needed are not furnished there can be no true counterpoise.

How do we expend the energy? By the common wear-and-tear incident upon all voluntary motion, all work and recreation, carrying on the internal movements of digestion and respiration, by thinking, by loss of temperature, by indulgence of any of our functions, and by any wrong indulgence especially. Excessive use, voluntary or otherwise, will of course diminish our total capital and cut short our lives. Could we always maintain the right balance we need never die.

The importance of what has been said must now be clearly apparent. We ought to be wisely interested in choosing the proper foods for our daily needs and in having them properly prepared; we ought to know how much carbohydrates we need, how much proteids, and regulate our diet accordingly. The foods which contain nitrogen are chiefly the following: flesh of all animals, milk, eggs, leguminous fruits (peas, beans, lentils); those which contain carbohydrates chiefly are bread, starch, vegetables and especially potatoes, rice, etc.; foods supplying fat are butter, lard, fat of meat, etc. Salts are furnished in almost all other substances, but especially in green vegetables and fruits. Liquid food is obtained by water, too often neglected, and tea, coffee, beer, cider, etc.

Alcohol has no power to form tissue or to repair waste and cannot be regarded as a true food. Tea and coffee are almost entirely stimulant, not nutritious, and should be taken sparingly or not at all.

The common mistakes in diet are over-feeding or taking too much of one kind of food, and of the latter class perhaps an excess of starchy food is the most mischievous. If taken in excess, especially by the young, the starchy foods are not digested and what does not digest must putrefy: the result is a bowel distended with harmful gases. Many people eat too much nitrogenous food, with resulting plethora or gout. A great deal of vigorous exercise in the open air is required to use up such a diet.

CHAPTER XXVIII.

SELECTION AND PREPARATION OF FOOD.

The requirements for normal digestion, assimilation and elimination are: (1) An intestinal canal clean and sound from mouth to anus; (2) nutritious food properly prepared; (3) regularity and moderation in eating; (4) free use of pure water, sufficient to forward the emulsification and assimilation of the food and the elimination of waste--whether that waste be of the residual portion of the food or of detritus of tissue; (5) a seasonably clad body, free from fatigue or loss of sleep; (6) a cheerful mind.

Every sensible person will grant that a good digestion of vegetable or animal food furnishes sufficient steam and stimulus for the physical man; that a good digestion of intellectual food (ideas) furnishes the corresponding requisites for the mental man; and that exalted sentiments are the pabulum of the spiritual.

Why over-stimulate the physical, and reflexively degrade the mental and spiritual, by indulgence in tea, coffee, beer, wine, liquors, opium, tobacco, etc.? Over-stimulation will bring on indigestion; and prostration will follow that. Remember that Nature does not carry long credit accounts.

A suggestion for the selection and preparation of physical foods is here given; this book being hardly the place for a corresponding list of mental and spiritual foods.

FOODS EASY OF DIGESTION.

ARTICLES OF FOOD HOW PREPARED TIME OF DIGESTION

Venison steak Broiled 1 hour 30 minutes Pig's feet soused Boiled 1 " 00 "

Brains Boiled 1 " 45 " Salmon, tripe or trout (fresh) Boiled or fried 1 " 00 " Eggs, fresh Whipped 1 " 30 " Rice Boiled 1 " 00 " Sago or barley Boiled 1 " 45 " Apples, sweet and mellow Raw 1 " 30 " Tomatoes or lettuce Raw 1 " 30 " Melons or watercress Raw 1 " 20 " Peaches, plums or pears Raw or stewed 1 " 30 " Oranges or bananas Raw 1 " 30 " Asparagus or dandelion Boiled 1 " 30 " Onions or apricots Stewed 1 " 30 " Mushrooms Boiled 1 " 30 " Cereal coffee Boiled 1 " 30 " Blackberries 1 " 30 " Grape-nuts 1 " 00 " Lemons 1 " 00 " Watermelons 1 " 00 " Doxsee's clam juice and little neck clams 1 " 00 " Milkine, Horlick's and Mellin's food 1 " 30 " Cereal milk 1 " 00 " Armour & Co.'s Vigoral. 1 " 00 " Valentine's or Wyeth's beef juice or Wiel's beef jelly 1 " 00 "

FOODS NOT SO EASY OF DIGESTION.

ARTICLES OF FOOD HOW PREPARED TIME OF DIGESTION

Beef Boiled 2 hours 00 minutes Pig, sucking Roasted 2 " 30 " Liver, beef (fresh) Broiled 2 " 00 " Lamb, fresh Broiled 2 " 30 " Turkey, domestic Roasted or boiled 2 " 30 " " wild Roasted 2 " 18 " Goose " Roasted 2 " 30 " Chicken Fricasseed 2 " 45 " Codfish, cured and dry Boiled 2 " 00 " Oysters, fresh Raw 2 " 35 " Hash (chopped meat and vegetables) Warmed 2 " 30 " Eggs, fresh Roasted 2 " 15 " " " Raw 2 " 00 " Milk Boiled 2 " 00 " " " Uncooked 2 " 15 " Gelatine Boiled 2 " 30 " Custard Baked 2 " 45 " Tapioca or barley Boiled 2 " 00 " Beans, green Boiled 2 " 30 " Sponge cake Baked 2 " 30 " Apples, sour and mellow Raw 2 " 00 " " " " " hard Raw 2 " 50 " Parsnips or green corn Boiled 2 " 30 " Potatoes and yams Roasted or baked 2 " 30 " Cabbage, head Raw 2 " 30 " " " with vinegar Raw 2 " 00 " Cauliflower Boiled 2 " 00 " Peas (green) or squash Boiled 2 " 00 " Cranberries or cherries Stewed 2 " 00 " Rhubarb or figs Stewed 2 " 30 " Turnips Boiled 2 " 30 " Sprouts Boiled 2 " 00 " Raspberries Raw 2 " 00 " Dates Raw 2 " 00 " Buttermilk Raw 2 " 00 " Pumpkin Cooked 2 " 00 "

FOODS SOMEWHAT DIFFICULT OF DIGESTION.

ARTICLES OF FOOD HOW PREPARED TIME OF DIGESTION

Beef, fresh, lean Broiled 3 hours 00 minutes " " " Roasted 3 " 00 " Beef, dry Roasted 3 " 30 " " with salt only Boiled 3 " 45 " " " mustard, etc. Boiled 3 " 30 " Pork, steak Broiled 3 " 15 " " recently salted Broiled 3 " 15 " " " " Raw 3 " 00 " " " " Stewed 3 " 00 " Mutton, fresh Broiled 3 " 00 " " " Roasted 3 " 15 " " " Boiled 3 " 00 " Flounder, fresh Boiled 3 " 30 " Oysters, fresh Roasted 3 " 15 " " " Stewed 3 " 30 " Codfish (salted) or whitefish Boiled 3 " 00 " Sausages, fresh Broiled 3 " 20 " Rabbits Broiled 3 " 00 " Butter or cream 3 " 00 " Eggs, fresh Hard-boiled or fried 3 " 30 " " " Soft-boiled 3 " 00 " Potatoes, turnips or carrots Boiled 3 " 30 " Radishes or lentils Boiled 3 " 30 " Bread (white) fresh Baked 3 " 15 " " whole wheat Baked 3 " 30 " " rye Baked 3 " 30 " " graham Baked 3 " 30 " " corn Baked 3 " 15 " Corn cake Baked 3 " 00 " Apple dumpling Boiled 3 " 00 " Soup, mutton or oyster Boiled 3 " 30 " " bean Boiled 3 " 00 " " chicken Boiled 3 " 00 " Chocolate or cocoa Boiled 3 " 00 " Currants or filberts 3 " 00 " Raisins 3 " 00 " Hazelnuts 3 " 30 " Peanuts Roasted 3 " 00 " Potatoes (sweet) Roasted 3 " 00 " Walnuts 3 " 30 " Chestnuts Roasted 3 " 15 " Beans, lima Boiled 3 " 00 " Zwieback 3 " 00 " Turkey Boiled or roasted 3 to 4 hours Eels Fried 3 " 4 " Oleomargarine 3 " 4 " Cabbage Boiled 3 " 4 " Buckwheat cakes 3 " 4 " Mutton, lean Roasted 3 " 4 " Herring Broiled 3-1/2 " 4-1/2 " Cheese 3-1/2 " 6 "

FOODS VERY DIFFICULT OF DIGESTION.

ARTICLES OF FOOD HOW PREPARED TIME OF DIGESTION

Beef, fresh, lean Fried 4 hours 00 minutes " old, hard, salted Boiled 4 " 15 " " recently salted Boiled 4 " 30 " " " " Fried 4 " 15 " " fat or lean Roasted 5 " 15 " " suet (fresh) Boiled 5 " 30 " " soup with vegetables and bread Boiled 4 " 00 " Beef, soup from marrow bones Boiled 4 " 15 " Pork, fat and lean Roasted 5 " 15 " " recently salted Boiled 4 " 00 " Pork recently salted Fried 4 " 15 " " ham Cured 4 " 30 " Veal Broiled 4 " 00 " " Fried 4 " 30 " Mutton, suet Boiled 4 " 30 " Fowls Boiled or roasted 4 " 00 " Heart, animal Fried 4 " 00 " Salmon, salted, or mackerel Boiled 4 " 00 " Cabbage, with vinegar Boiled 4 " 30 " Cheese, old, strong Raw 3-1/2 to 6-1/2 hours Duck Roasted 4 hours 30 "

CHAPTER XXIX.

DIET FOR INDIGESTION.

Indigestion is a symptom of a functional disturbance or is due to a local disease in some portion of the digestive apparatus. Therefore diet must be adapted to the sensibility of the stomach and bowels, to gastric and intestinal secretions, mobility, absorption and elimination, to the abnormal increased feeling of hunger or to the absence of the sensation of hunger.

The food should be of easy solubility and offer slight resistance to the digestive juices. It should not mechanically or chemically irritate or impede intestinal peristalsis. It should not increase fermentation or putrefaction and the greater portion of it should be absorbed.

The object of diet is not to eat less food than usual but to secure more nourishment until the proper quantity is consumed each day. The restriction of foods does not mean limitation. Regular hours for meals should be religiously observed by sufferers from indigestion. The food should be thoroughly masticated. Good judgment should be used by each individual in selecting and preparing the foodstuffs; also in the amount taken at each meal, and the proper length of time to continue the diet.

You may take:

Soup--in moderate quantity: Doxsee's clam juice, and little neck clams; cream of peas, etc.; vermicelli; tapioca; tomato; clear soups of chicken, beef, mutton.

Fish: trout; bass; perch; shad; weakfish; whitefish; smelts; raw oysters.

Meat: roasted or boiled beef; mutton; venison; calf s head; tongue;

sweetbread; lamb chops; squab; roasted partridge; pigeon; calf's-foot jelly; Armour & Co.'s Vigoral; Valentine's or Wyeth's beef juice, or Wiel's beef jelly.

Eggs: raw; soft-boiled; poached; omelette; eggs on toast.

Bread--all over a day old: brown; graham; gluten; rye; zwieback; crackers; cracked wheat; corn meal; hominy; wheaten and graham grits; rolled rye and oats; granose; cerealin; macaroni with toasted bread-crumbs; farina, boiled with milk; Milkine; Horlick's or Mellin's food.

Vegetables: spinach; green peas; greens; lettuce; watercress; sweet corn; asparagus; celery; artichokes; baked tomatoes; cauliflower.

Dessert: baked, roasted or stewed apples; stewed pears or peaches; baked bananas; grapes; oranges; and most ripe fruits, if fresh.

Beverages: hot, cool or cold water an hour before meals. Drink freely of the same during meal-time, but not to wash down food. Drink also: cereal coffee; buttermilk; koumiss; fresh cider; bouillon.

Avoid: coffee; tea; milk; ice-water; cocoa; chocolate; malt liquors; spirituous liquors; sweet and effervescent wines; sugar; candies; foods containing much starch; rich soups; sauces and chowders; all fried foods; hot or fresh bread; griddle-cakes; doughnuts; veal; pork; liver; kidney; hashes; stews; pickled, canned, preserved and potted meats; turkey; goose; duck; sausage; salmon; salt mackerel; cabbage; radishes; cucumbers; cole-slaw; turnips: potatoes; beets; pastry; jellies; jams; nuts.

CHAPTER XXX.

DIET FOR CONSTIPATION AND OBSTIPATION.

Diet is too often a makeshift for ignorance, or it may be an aid until the cause of indigestion is removed; or if not curable, a compromise effected on the best possible terms for continued existence. We have found out the almost universal cause for constipation, obstipation and costiveness; therefore until you can have the proper local treatment we suggest the following foodstuffs, trusting to the sufferer's judgment how much and how often to take the nourishment.

Coarse foods, stimulants and laxatives unduly excite the bowels. Avoid them if possible. Be regular in your habits as to meal-times; eat three times daily, and about an equal amount at each meal.

You may take:

Soup: all kinds of meat and vegetable soup; broth; bouillon. Reliable preparations of beef juice, jelly, etc.

Fish: all kinds, broiled or baked; raw oysters; Doxsee's clam preparations.

Meat: boiled or roasted; poultry; game, etc.

Bread: graham; brown; whole wheat; corn; rye; ginger; shredded-wheat biscuit.

Cereals: wheaten grits; wheatena; granose; oatmeal porridge; Milkine; Horlick's and Mellin's food.

Vegetables: cauliflower; spinach; beans; asparagus; carrots; onions; Brussels sprouts; tomatoes; peas; celery; cabbage.

Vegetables should be especially well cooked to render them soft and easy of digestion.

Salads: may be eaten if dressed with a generous supply of olive oil.

Dessert: oranges; melons; prunes; tamarinds; figs; apples (raw or baked);

pears; plums; peaches; cherries; raisins; stewed fruit; honey; blackberries; strawberries; huckleberries; bananas.

Some may find it advantageous to eat fruit before or between meals.

Beverages: water--pure spring water preferably; if this cannot be had, get, if possible, distilled water that has been agitated; buttermilk; fresh cider; beer; ale.

Mineral waters like Hunyadi, etc., irritate the cause of constipation (proctitis) in a way similar to cathartic remedies.

Drink a tumbler or more of hot or cold water an hour before meals-- preferably hot water. If the hot water be distasteful add a little salt. Drink freely of water about the temperature of 60?during the meals, but not for the purpose of emptying the mouth of food.

On retiring at night and rising in the morning sip slowly from a quarter to half pint of water (hot or cold). In the morning be sure to rinse the mouth free of the accumulated mucus before drinking the water.

The use of tea, chocolate, coffee and alcoholic drinks is so abused by those even who consider themselves temperate in their habits, that I recommend these beverages as remedies only in certain conditions of the system.

About four pints of pure water (i.e., free from all salts or other foreign ingredients) should be imbibed in twenty-four hours.

Avoid: sweets; pastry of all kinds; puddings; rice; milk; cheese; new bread; nuts; fried foods; rich gravies; farina and sago puddings; salt meats; salt fish; veal; goose; liver; hard-boiled eggs; pork; tea; tobacco; spirituous liquors; uncooked strawberries and huckleberries. Avoid also tomatoes and peaches when not fresh, as the acid generated by keeping them a few days is very irritating to an already inflamed bowel.

Avoid substances that would inflame the tissues or cause congestion of any organ of the body. If the tongue be coated avoid sugar, starchy foods and fresh milk.

CHAPTER XXXI.

COSTIVENESS, DIET, ETC.

Take anything in the way of food which the unconsciously starved person can eat without the stomach and intestines protesting too much; any of the foods recommended for constipation, indigestion, diarrhea; and take yet more food if by so doing there is a gain in flesh, after exercising much patience as to time.

Irrigate the system by imbibing freely of hot and cold water at various periods of the day. Good red wine mixed with the water drunk at meal-time may serve a good purpose in helping to enrich the blood.

Keep the pores of the skin open by bathing; and all the functions of the body active by exercise, massage, pure air, sunlight, rest, sleep and seasonable clothing.

The large intestines should be kept clean by proper amounts of water injected into them. The local cause of all the trouble should be treated by a competent physician.

And with all the efforts, continue the treatment long enough to accomplish some good and then a much longer time to get well. Do not give up treatment under which you have improved if it requires one, two or three years to accomplish what you have so well started out to do.

CHAPTER XXXII.

DIET FOR DIARRHEA.

A period marked by constipation, biliousness or poisons generated within or taken into the intestinal canal is often followed by diarrhea. Mental excitement will induce it in some persons. More often man's early and most common malady, proctitis, is the direct or indirect cause. Some forms of ulceration of the lower bowel induce diarrhea. Chronic cases of diarrhea usually follow the decline of vitality marked by the symptom of Costiveness, which means the interruption of all the functions of nutrition. The intestinal canal is then like a rubber tube with the contents hurried through it. The whole system is irritable as the result of an accumulation of secondary symptoms expressed by the word auto-intoxication.

The food should be nutritious and non-irritating to the intestinal canal.

Reliance must be placed, in severe cases, on liquid foods and beverages.

The more solid foods may be taken in limited quantity as the recovery progresses. In more acute cases it is well to stop all food for twelve or twenty-four hours.

You may take:

Liquid Food and Beverages: Drink, if possible, pure spring water. If this cannot be obtained, sterilize the water, or distil and agite it; it must be pure and soft. Better still: drink toast- or rice-water; kefyr, four days old; koumiss; lactic-acid water; zoolak; egg lemonade; sterilized milk with one third lime-water; whortleberry wine; acorn cocoa; unfermented grape-juice.

Soup: chicken; mutton; clam; oyster broth; Doxsee's clam-juice; bouillon; Milkine; Horlick's and Mellin's food.

Meat: minced chicken; scraped beef; roast fowl; beef steak; fillet of beef; raw beef; sweetbread; raw oysters.

Eggs: lightly boiled, poached.

Cereals and Fruit: grapes at all hours, eaten without seeds or skin; arrowroot; tapioca; sago; barley mush; macaroni; rice boiled with milk; milk toast; dry toast; crackers; junket; bread pudding; egg pudding, not sweetened; hasty pudding, with flour and milk; mashed potatoes.

Avoid: pork; veal; nuts; salt meats; fish; fried foods; sugary foods; fruits, cooked or raw; oatmeal; brown and graham bread; new bread; vegetables; and most soups.

A FINAL WORD TO THOSE TO WHOM I HAVE DEDICATED THIS BOOK.

It is very evident from the perusal of this work that the symptoms of proctitis, both general and local, proceed from no trifling disease; and also that the disease may have existed for a very long time, perhaps as much as twenty, forty or more years. During the greater part of its existence all sorts of medication have been tried to allay this or that annoying prominent symptom with a hope of a cure.

At the congress of physicians that met in Paris in 1900, one of the subjects discussed was chronic constipation and their "wise" conclusion was that man needed more grease, therefore they mourned the loss of the frying-pan.

Symptoms induced by proctitis in various parts of the body are often accompanied by painful local symptoms, called piles or a "touch of the piles." Then local medication is added to the general treatment, and as usual matters go from bad to worse. Physicians consulted have been honest and kind, but with all their advice the increasing troubles continue. Your demands grow more pressing on your doctor and as a last resort he mentions a surgical operation for the removal of one or more painful local symptoms. The fright is sufficient in most cases to make the sufferer endure the ills he has rather than flee to others he knows not, even risking life itself. Others more bold submit to an examination by the surgeon, which proves so painful at the time and causes so much subsequent suffering that they are now really content not to importune any more for help.

A few in desperation make up their minds to have the local anal symptom removed regardless of the final result.

Thus millions of human beings have suffered and died and countless numbers are enduring the ills they have, not knowing of a rational and humane system of treatment; a treatment that not only removes the numerous annoying symptoms, but the cause as well; a system that will stand the test of time, of common-sense, of constant investigation to know the why and wherefore of both disease and treatment.

For over twenty years I have concerned myself with this and allied ailments, and have treated--without the use of the knife--all cases of piles, polypus, fissure, stricture, ulcerations, etc. At the present time physicians are writing me in this wise: "I want to take a course of instruction from you. I have performed some successful surgical operations on the rectum, but it is not profitable; the people will not submit to it." Another writes: "Your treatment of hemorrhoids has been brought to my notice by my friend and patient, Mr. ----. The method you practise is certainly an ideal one and seems to have been most successful in your hands, and I would like to adopt it."

To physicians and laymen interested, I will send, for twenty-five cents, my treatise on Diseases of the Anus and Rectum (entitled How to Become Strong). It contains over 100 anatomical illustrations, and 125 testimonials, and forms, therefore, a valuable adjunct to this volume.

All whose testimonials appear in the 64-page book suffered from proctitis to a greater or less extent and with the exception of a few all suffered from chronic constipation, indigestion, etc.

Surgeons usually desire strong and vigorous patients. The author asks merely for an intelligent patient, or for some one to direct the home attention necessary between treatments.

This book, as well as the one entitled How to Become Strong, and the author's other printed instructions, are the result of his desire to make his patients intelligent on the subject of the disease and symptoms for which they seek his assistance. They truly cannot know too much for their own good in this regard; an ignorant patient can not do justice either to himself or to his physician. Those who have tried all the fads and so-called cures in order to relieve their troubles will certainly appreciate what I have here presented for their study. With enlightenment comes the desire to set things right. So I have no appeal to make to the lazy: I shall leave them to their ills and their pills. And for those who appreciate the beauty of cleanliness, both external and internal, I shall write another book on that subject, including a prophecy for coming generations. Eternal vigilance is the price we must pay if we would enjoy the highest physical, mental and spiritual expression of our personalities.

Thanking the indulgent reader who has read my description of Intestinal Ills, I advise him to rewrite it in his own organism, if not in printer's ink: the world will be better for it!

INTESTINAL ILLS.

NO. 1.

CHRONIC CONSTIPATION AND THE USE OF THE ENEMA.

"Civilized" man is the victim, by inheritance from distant ancestors, of undesirable characteristics, traits, and tendencies. While, during the long process of evolution, some of the cruder features of the physical and mental traits have been refined or eliminated, the modern man still clings to certain habits inherited from his wholly animalistic days. Even as the man of that day, so the man of to-day eats far too much and far too frequently.

To the scientific eye, your capacious digestive apparatus is a psycho-physical exhibit of the racial proclivity to overeat. Here, in this exhibit, the race's inordinate craving for food and drink, its gluttonous thought, have embodied themselves; and this exhibit, this apparatus, is accordingly not merely physical, but also psychical, for its sub-conscious outreach for "more and always more" is only too apparent. Man's stomach and bowels are too much like those of a mere animal, and are the source of nine-tenths of his ills.

All great consumers of foodstuffs, Nature declares, should walk on all fours; if you will persist in walking on your hind legs, you will have to pay the penalty. You will, moreover, contract other habits not conducive to real animal health. And, as Nature predicted, man's social customs to-day are out of all accord with gluttonous feeding; he, as well as his capacious bowels, suffers the consequences of his excessive feeding, and this suffering leads him to adopt artificial means for relief or escape. Up-to-date civilization has constrained man to adopt a cooped-up existence, one that shuts out, to a great extent, sunshine and air; an existence, moreover, that involves but a limited amount of exercise. How, then, can it be otherwise than--gormand that he is--that he should fare ill with this gluttonous, mammoth digestive canal?

Man is not as yet more than half human, and he will not become truly human until he makes more use of the upper lobes of his brain, nor until the spiritual part of his nature becomes dominant. When that day dawns he will have a corresponding evolution of the physical body, especially of the gastro-intestinal canal. Some one has sagely said that man's brain is a mere extension of his intestinal canal. Well, possibly by and by the intestinal canal may become an extension of a spiritually awakened mind, with all its dominating influence over the physical body. Surely the evolutional trend from animal to complete manhood may be aided by intelligent foresight as to bodily care and hygiene.

Cooped up like a canary bird, or penned up and fattening like a hog, with his enormous eating capacity and vast intestinal storage space, poor man has matters made worse by having his several orifices liable to inflammatory invasions. He does not seem able to escape from his enemies anywhere.

The mucous membrane lining the orifices of the body is nothing more than the skin turned in to line canals for air, gases, liquids, and solids to pass in and out in order to keep up the physio-logical functions of the body. Very rarely, indeed, do we find, from childhood to old age, the orifice of the intestinal sewer otherwise than chronically inflamed, the invasion extending, moreover, the whole length of the rectum for some distance into the sigmoid colon.

It is no trifling matter to have the function of some thirty feet of the gastro-intestinal tract disturbed, especially of the large intestine--some five feet in length, two and a half inches in diameter in not a few sections.

Almost without exception, we find the lower portion of the intestinal sewer the seat of chronic inflammation that extends into the sigmoid colon; and, as an inevitable result of the inflammation, contraction more or less permanent has taken place in the circular and longitudinal muscular bands that form its structure. The constriction is especially severe at the junction of the rectum with the sigmoid colon, where it flexes upon itself in the region where the bore of the rectum is less. The comparative shutting up of the caliber of the upper end of the rectum and lower portion of the sigmoid colon occasions undue retention of the feces and gases which accumulate, and in accumulating dislocate various portions of the large intestine, thus forming pouches, sacks, reservoirs, prolapse, etc., which hold the products of putrefaction as well as the irritating, poisonous mucus thrown out from the inflamed tissue.

I regard the occlusion of the upper portion of the rectum, and especially of the region involved in the flexure of the bowel, as the most usual seat and source of constipation. Not so very long ago it was the custom to stretch the sphincter muscles for the "cure" of constipation; at the present time the "cure" is found in the valves of the middle lower portion of the rectum. The folly of these "cures" becomes apparent when we understand that the parts treated were neither the seat nor the source of constipation. I have always regarded great retention of feces in the rectum as impaction in a delivery canal, due to contraction of the anal muscles, not as constipation, which can only take place in the temporary storage-place--the sigmoid flexure. The lower two-thirds of the rectum plays no part in constipation of the bowels.

Form a manikin, made out of very thin, soft rubber tubing, to represent the stomach and small and large intestine, holding the various parts in place with elastic bands, and cotton to represent fat. When all portions are properly and anatomically placed close the lower eight or ten inches of the manikin, representing the lower portion of the sigmoid colon, rectum, and anus, just as tightly as we should find it closed in sufferers from chronically acute proctitis and colitis. Now insert at the stomach portion of the manikin a generous amount of man's usual mixture of foodstuffs and liquids, and repeat the supply three or four times during the day (without any previous attempts at cleansing), and then note the fermentative and putrefactive changes that take place; the ensuing bacterial poisons and the great volume of poisonous gases--all of which occasion squirming, twisting movements of the manikin as dislocations here and there occur, as pouches and reservoirs develop, as the walls become distended with gas and putrid substance; and then, time elapsing, the usual foodstuffs are added to the foul mass within! Now, if there is any pity in your soul, you medical man, for the enfouled and deformed human manikin, you will want to wash it out with cleansing water before its structure comes to an untimely end. We medical men all know the numerous and grave symptoms exhibited by one or more organs of the body, or by all of them, from the persistent work of the deleterious gases and bacterial poisons on the system--a work going on for years, finally placing the victim beyond medical aid. All of us are agreed that the capacious gastro-intestinal canal should be clean. What, I submit, is the best means of keeping clean this long, large, tortuous, spacious, valved and flexed canal--a canal that disease has here and there pouched, dislocated, bagged, reservoired; a canal at whose lower end a great cesspool exists; that, like other portions of the gut, is never empty and clean--what is the best means but a flushing with copious amount of water?

Proctitis or colitis is a very serious disease; like a railroad injury, it is found, on examination, to be much worse than appearances at first indicated.

A physician who prescribes for a case of chronic constipation or diarrhea without first examining the sufferer for proctitis and colitis, is either ignorant or does wilful harm to his patient and injury to his practice. The abominable, aboriginal and almost universal custom at the present time of giving some physic to "cleanse" the gastro-intestinal canal is in every respect a deplorable mistake for a conscientious doctor to make.

Many persons suffering from chronic constipation drink very little or no water. As a consequence, they are a sort of dirty, dried-up plant, with but little juice of life in them.

Others, again, equally unclean, or more so, take a moderate amount of fluid every day, and present a more or less roly-poly appearance, with considerable abdominal distention, due to malnutrition and gases. Of course, their eyes, skin, tongue, breath, and lack of vim and vigor tell the story of a long process of self-poisoning, with every now and then the eventuation of a storm of foulness, called a bilious attack--meaning an overflow of filth. Death often brings about a radical change in such poisoned bodies.

Now, what can a prescriber of a gastro-intestinal ejector expect to accomplish by disturbing the maleconomy of this apparatus? Usually he expects that considerable trouble will ensue; consequently, he will add belladonna or some other soothing drug to mitigate the act of expulsion. The ejector (called laxative, purgative, cathartic) occasions irritation, which sets up twisting, writhing, rumbling of the bowels, accompanied with a shower of liquid into the canal (as tears fill the eyes from the effects of sand or a blow), which liquid mingles again with the putrid refuse materials, from which it had been recently absorbed, and, mingling, proceeds to fill up the normal and abnormal spaces just described, to be again reabsorbed into the system. Oh, the foulness of it all! The spirits of the departed, as well as the still incarnate patients, demand of the healing art safe and sane hygienic methods of cure. The enema, regularly and properly used, is the remedy par excellence.

Those that suffer from chronic constipation are usually deficient in the quantity and quality of intestinal secretions. Physic increases the depletion of the intestinal juices. Of the watery secretion forced into the bowels, four-fifths are reabsorbed into the system, plus poisons and filth. The system soon becomes accustomed to the irritation of drugs, and requires an ever-increasing amount. These irritate and increase the chronic inflammation of the lower bowel, often to the extent of a discharge of blood.

Straining effort to induce defecation is injurious. The use of massage, of vibratory exercises, of electricity; the spraying of cold water on the abdomen, etc.,--none of them are calculated to remove or even to relieve the proctitis and colitis.

The temperature of the water used for an enema should be about one hundred degrees. It should be taken at least twice daily, preferably on retiring at night and soon after breakfast, at regular times, if possible. Such practice obviates the need of large injections.

In beginning the use of the enema it is well to inject from a half to a pint of water, and expel it. This constitutes a preliminary injection. Frequently it is desirable to take another preliminary injection before taking the large one, which latter is variously called "flushing the colon," "taking an enema," "taking an internal bath" or "a washout," etc. It is essential first to get rid of the feces and gases in the rectum, so that they be not sent back when you proceed to flush the colon.

NO. 2.

OBJECTIONS TO THE USE OF ENEMA ANSWERED.

The privilege of raising objections belongs to the ignorant as well as to the intelligent. But the objector is under as great obligations to state his reasons as the advocate.

The first plausible objection to the use of the enema is that it is not natural.

Admitting this charge, I should say that, inasmuch as proctitis, colitis, and constipation are unnatural, the use of a preternatural or, in other words, a rational means to overcome the consequences of these diseases is imperative. The enema is such a means.

Can any one that suffers from proctitis, etc., have a natural stool? Unnatural conditions require preternatural aids, as we all know. The injected water dilates the constricted portion of the gut and arouses a revulsive impulse to expel the invading water. In obeying this impulse the imprisoned feces, gases, etc., are ejected with the water.

It may be unnatural to put water into the rectum, etc., but once there its expulsion from healthy bowels would be quite natural. No natural action can be expected from unhealthy bowels; they do the best they can under the circumstances. Eye-glasses, false teeth, crutches, etc., are unnatural but invaluable aids, but no more so than is the enema as a means of relief from overloaded bowels. The enema, moreover, be it noted, not only aids the system by relieving it of its loads; it cleanses and soothes an organ that must be kept at work and perform its functions even when invaded by disease.

Surely it is unhygienic and irrational to ignore the valuable service of the enema in cases in which the bowels are in an unnatural condition.

The second objection is that the water will wash away the mucus from the mucous membrane of the bowels and leave them dry and parched, and thus apt to crack and break in two. I would remind the objector that, since about 75 per cent. of the normal feces is water, it seems strange that so great a quantity of water in contact with the mucous surface of the bowels should not also cause dryness.

The integument of the body and that of the mucous membrane are similar in structure, yet whoever had a fear of producing dryness of the skin by much application of water? The mucous membrane is simply the skin turned inward; and since it is much more vascular it is less apt to become dry--if, indeed, its dryness were at all possible. The objector should also remember that the body is composed of over 80 per cent. of water--an organism not to be made dry or parched by the application of water to the skin or to the mucous membrane two or three times a day.

The mucous membrane of the lower bowel is not unlike that of the mouth, throat, or stomach. Do you realize how often the upper end of the intestinal canal is washed or bathed daily with liquids, soft and hard drinks, hot and cold, especially by those who have formed the drink habit instead of the enema habit?

They have no fear of drying the mucous membrane thereby; but if you can instil this fear they will increase the quantity with pleasure.

This second objection, being the result of too vivid an imagination and too little reflection, is a very nonsensical objection indeed.

A third objection is that if you begin the use of the enema you will have to continue its use; you can't stop, and, lo and behold! the enema habit is formed--a new habit in addition to the many habits civilized man is already carrying; the constipated habit, the physic habit, the sand, bran, sawdust-food habit, the muscular peristaltic habit, etc.--and with all these habits the poor victim of proctitis and intestinal foulness wonders that he is alive.

Usually the first symptom of proctitis is constipation, and for relief the enema habit should be formed and continued while the constipation remains. When the proper means are found to remove the intestinal inflammation--proctitis and colitis--then the constipation will disappear, and with its disappearance the enema habit can be discontinued. But let it be well noted that the enema is itself an aid in curing the cause, an aid superior to any other at our command. A cleanly habit ought not to be an objectionable one, especially in cases in which it is most needed to prevent toxic substances from entering the system.

A fourth objection is that after taking the first enema the constipation is worse.

With many persons a certain amount of undue accumulation of feces will excite a sufficient muscular effort of the gut to force the dried mass through the proctitis- and colitis-strictured bowels. This unnatural effort may occur once a day or once in two or three days, and has doubtless been a habit of many years' duration.

To introduce a new order of conduct on the part of the bowels requires time. If the bowels have been in the habit of expelling feces in the morning, and an enema were taken the night before, there might be no desire to stool the next morning because of the fact that the bulk or accumulated mass of excrement was no longer there to create a vigorous call or impulse for defecation.

But we have found the extent of local damage and reflex to the organs, and more especially the constant absorption of poisons into the system, due to the presence of feces. It is for this reason that the elimination of feces twice or thrice in twenty-four hours is advised. The condition for which an enema is used is one of disturbance and poison to the system. It is, therefore, a most unnatural condition. What is more rational, consequently, than to employ an "unnatural" yet not harmful means to bring about a more normal condition, one free from poisoning and irritating consequences?

A fifth objection is made by those who have as a symptom of proctitis a large development of pile tumors or hemorrhoids (distended mucous membrane). The objection is that at times these tumors or sacs prolapse very freely during the act of expelling the injected water. But this prolapse occurs in many cases whether water is used or not.

A certain amount of anal irritation caused by the passage of feces occurs, causing contraction of the circular muscular tissue that forms the anal and rectal canal, also of the longitudinal muscular bands and the levator muscles of the organs. The enema lessens or entirely diminishes the irritation of passing feces, and the natural result is that the serum-filled sacs, called piles, and the tissue loosened by the inflammatory product will more readily prolapse during the act of defecating. It is simply a choice between irritation of the stool keeping the tissue up and no irritation permitting a prolapse.

Of course, if there be no expulsion of feces and water the stretched or dilated sacs may keep their places in the rectum. And then again, the enema may be used for quite a period, when all at once a large prolapse of sacculated mucous membrane occurs, and the enema is thought to be the cause of it. That this is not the cause, let it be remembered that in all cases of proctitis the chronic inflammation is apt to become subacute or acute, and that this intense engorgement and enlargement of the tissue with blood and the increased fever in the parts often result in prolapse at any time, especially at times of convulsive effort at evacuation.

Whatever follows the proper use of an enema, even though what follows be annoying, should not be blamed on the enema, for its action is most kindly, lessening as it does the irritation that otherwise would be more severe when the feces pass through a disease-constricted canal.

The sixth objection is that the use of the enema will weaken the bowels, which are already too "weak" to expel their contents. "Atony, paralysis, fatty degeneration of the gut, are bad enough," say these objectors, "without having an enema increase their uselessness." Diagnosis wrong and objection groundless.

Distend and contract an organ for a short time two or three times a day, and it will gain in strength from the exercise. Every one knows that this is the case. What more gentle means of exercising the large intestines than by the enema?

But the truth of the matter is that in all cases of proctitis and constipation the diseased portion of the gut is too active in its muscular movements, contracting spasmodically, as it does, at even the suggestion or suspicion of feces near it. Every impulse of the bowels above the constricted section to force the feces down through the closed bore only intensifies the spasmodic action and increases the muscular obstruction, compelling the victim to resort to some one of the many drastic means of relief.

The enema does no more than kindly to dilate the constricted region, which, when dilated, evokes a harmonious concerted action of all the nerves and muscles to pass along and down the burden of feces, which, without the aid of a flood of water, they had been incapable of moving, and would have had to leave to poison the system.

The seventh objection is quite naive: "Inasmuch as the Indians of this country had no use for the enema, why should we resort to it?"

The all-sufficient answer to this objection is that the Indians lived a natural life, while ours is artificial. Much can be said on this point, but the reader is surely rational enough to follow out the distinction suggested. Our lives are much more important than were the lives of the aborigines of this country, and our "demands of Nature" are more exigent. If your life is of no greater value than theirs, for leisure's sake don't use the enema! You will be taking too much trouble. It really should seem that the cleanliness of the skin and mucous membrane, the care we take of our bodies, is an indication and measure of our sense of refinement. An ancient Scripture hath it: "Let those that are filthy, be filthy still." It all depends upon how you wish to be classed-- with the filthy or the cleanly.

The eighth objection to be noted is the fear of "poking things" (points of instruments) "into the rectum."

This looks like a real objection. No healthy nor even unhealthy organ, for that matter, should be "abused." And what seems more likely to cause it trouble than to poke a hard or soft rubber point or tube through its vent in opposition to its bent or inclination? Still, the muscles of the vent are strong, and they soon accommodate themselves to the practice. Their slight disinclination is not to be considered alongside of the relief and cure you effect by the use of the enema.

Have no fear that the point will occasion disease when intelligently used. Always see to it that the point is scrupulously clean. Those made of hard rubber or metal can be kept so without effort.

Soft rubber points are always foul and dangerous, especially after they are used a few times. A good rule is never to put a point higher in the bowel than is absolutely necessary.

The ninth objection seems serious. It is that in taking an enema the water escaping from the syringe point will injure the mucous membrane where the jet strikes. But on examination this objection falls to the ground, for it stands to reason the jet cannot directly hit the surface for more than a moment. Immediately thereafter the accumulation of water will force the jet to spend its energy on the increasing volume, to lift it out of the way so that the continuous inflow may find room.

But even were it possible for the jet to strike a definite section of the mucous membrane during the taking of the enema, it could do no harm provided the water be at the proper temperature. And this is true even if a hydrant pressure be used. Not a few persons use the hydrant pressure of their houses in taking an enema. For a really successful flushing of the colon a considerable pressure is requisite to force the volume up and along a distance of five feet, especially when sitting upright. But it is folly to use a long syringe point, since it is like introducing one canal into another for the purpose of cleansing it. Therefore, have no fear from the use of proper syringe points; the jet of water will not hurt the mucous membrane. My professional brethren at least ought to know that the idea of such harm is sheer nonsense.

The tenth objection to using an enema is in being obliged to use it from the fact of having such a disease as chronic inflammation of the rectum and colon. Every victim hates to be compelled to do a thing, and the victim of proctitis and colitis is no exception to the rule. In fact, he is beginning to realize that unless he uses it his system will be poisoned by the absorption of the sewage waste. Let the victim object to the disease that necessitates the use of the enema and he will shortly be well. Then this objection to the use of the enema will indeed be the most important of all.

The eleventh objection, and the most ridiculous of all, is that it requires too much time to take the enema twice or thrice daily.

I lose all patience with persons urging this objection. Those that have little or no system with their daily duties seldom have time to do anything of importance. They suffer from "haphazarditis," a very difficult disease to cure, and they are in many cases hopeless. Usually they are an uncleanly lot of people, full of good intentions, but their intentions though taken often, seldom operate as an antidote to foulness. Their one sigh the livelong day is: "Oh, could we be like birds that can stool while on the wing or on foot!" This feat of time-saving being hardly possible in the present incarnation and order of society, they content themselves with making a storehouse out of the intestinal canal for an indefinite length of time as they concern themselves with external affairs of work or sport. A sorry lot they are indeed when they are laid up for repairs. Many doctors, I am sorry to say, encourage with a chuckle this foolish practice. "Any time to stool you can manage to get, so that you stool at least once a day, or once in every two or three days; stool when it is normal for you to do so." This criminal advice just suits the sleepy, the lazy, or the "awfully busy."

The American habit of doing things en masse, of handling things in large quantities or in bulk, has something to do with their don't care constipated habit. Small evacuations two or three times a day seem too much like small business, which, of course, is a waste of precious time. Wholesaling, laziness, lack of system, hurry, are the cause of good-for-nothingness of body and mind. It should never be too much trouble to restore the lost impulse for stooling twice or thrice daily.

Is it a small matter to have the main sewer of a city partly or entirely closed, or the main sewer pipe of a dwelling stopped up? Think of the dire results, notwithstanding that the windows and doors remain wide open! The Board of Health would soon deal with the negligent official or landlord. With very few exceptions, "civilized" men, women, and children are negligent and niggardly caretakers of the human dwelling place--the marvellous body of man. "Lack of time," "haven't the time," or "no time," is the excuse they give themselves and others.

Notwithstanding the numberless victims around them, none of these negligent and niggardly ones seem to get alarmed until the secondary symptoms, such as indigestion, gout, rheumatism, or disease of some vital organ, are sufficiently annoying to demand attention. But I have full faith in humanity. Man does the best he knows how, as a general rule. But often he doesn't know how; he needs enlightening.

The hints I have given will, I am confident, be considered and acted upon by all to whose attention they are brought, for by acting upon them, normal bodies and minds will result, and blessings attained heretofore considered impossible. Normal health depends on right doing and being. Eternal vigilance is the price to be paid for the attainment and maintenance of the goal of normal life and progress. Eliminate all waste material from the body and all shifty vermin from the mind, and the millennium for all things in the universe will soon dawn.

FOURTEEN REASONS

WHY WE SHOULD BATHE INTERNALLY AS WELL AS EXTERNALLY

1. Because very few persons are free from chronic inflammation of the anus, rectum, and sigmoid flexure, which causes contraction of the caliber of the organs.

2. None escape self-poisoning from the gastro-intestinal canal. Many are constantly being poisoned from the entrance of bacterial and other toxic substances into the system.

3. Nine-tenths of the ills that afflict mankind have their origin in a foul digestive apparatus and a consequently poisoned body.

4. Disease of the anus, rectum, and sigmoid flexure results in from two-thirds to three-fourths of the feces being daily absorbed into the system.

5. Feces unduly retained become very foul or malodorous. If the feces of birds and domestic fowls and animals were as obnoxious as that usually ejected by man their discharges would require immediate removal from human neighborhoods.

6. Man is the only creature that has formed the habit of making a fecal cesspool of his large intestine; hence his diseases of many varieties. There is nothing wholesome about him and he is quite destitute of vim, vigor, and push. The fecal poisoning of his parents is stamped upon him, and the unhygienic condition of his bowels makes matters worse.

7. Man needs to form the habit of stooling as frequently as birds, fowls, and quadrupeds--at least as many times in twenty-four hours as he partakes of food.

8. Making a reservoir of the lower bowels is not a time-saving habit, but, on the contrary, a breeder of many poisons, causing all sorts of acute and chronic diseases, which demand much time and attention, as countless

numbers know to their sorrow.

9. You are a factor in the social and business world; then why not look, feel, and be your best by simply adopting internal hygienic measures?

10. By the use of the Internal J.B.L. Cascade Bath you can secure two or three stools a day, as desired; and while you are preventing self-poisoning you are regaining a normal habit and natural health, which for so many years and generations have been denied you. Do not longer perpetuate the dire results of a foul alimentary canal and consequently diseased body.

11. All desire to be strong and healthy, and many would add beauty of form and complexion, which is also commendable. This can be attained by preventing disease through hygienic attention and the proper use of water.

12. The gastro-intestinal canal is a physiological, moving food supply for the body, and, like any other vessel that has contained fermenting substances, it should be emptied and cleaned before a fresh supply is put into it. This is only a sensible, reasonable, and cleanly duty to one's self.

13. Who can fear being made sick by adopting cleanly habits? You have perhaps tried all other means to keep well, and have failed; now try intestinal cleanliness--a method you should have thought of long ago.

14. Every one desires to avoid surgery, the taking of numerous medicines, and the spending of money in that way--and they can be avoided if you keep clean, both internally and externally.

* * * * *

www.ingramcontent.com/pod-product-compliance
Lightning Source LLC
Chambersburg PA
CBHW070323190526
45169CB00005B/1717